Crying in the Shower
Cervical Cancer

by
Pamela Ayer

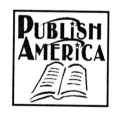

PublishAmerica

Baltimore

ISBN: 1-4137-6995-0
PUBLISHED BY PUBLISHAMERICA, LLLP
www.publishamerica.com
Baltimore

Printed in the United States of America

Dedication

This book is dedicated to my new husband, Jim King.
He is my Cowboy and my Texan

Without his encouragement, I would have never attempted
to write this book.

He gave me the courage to tell my story, and express all
of the emotions that I have hidden throughout my life
and during my struggle with cancer

To you Dear Cowboy, I say Thank you.

I Love You

Introduction

I step into my shower to wash away the tears,

For I cannot show my family, that I am filed with fears.

Doctors say that I have Cancer, and they'll try and get it all,

Is it too late to tell you, how much I love you all?

It is not what you have lost that is important.

It is what you already have, and take for granted.

Pamela Ayer
10/19/1999

Foreword

This is my true story. It spans only a short eight months of my life. It is an all to familiar story of the disease Cancer and its effect on the family and ones self.

The lessons which I learned from this experience, I wanted and needed to share. My wish is for anyone who should read this, will gather strength and hope from my victory.

Whether or not I shall stay Cancer free is not known. I can only keep my faith and take each day and live it to the best of my ability and be thankful for the extra time God has allowed me.

I wish for anyone fighting their own battle, whether it is with an illness or some other form of pain....to never give up.

There can be a tomorrow.

Chapter 1
The Beginning

It was a quarter to twelve, and there were only a few minutes before my visit to the doctor. I had been so nervous that morning that I wasn't sure if I had completed all my duties for the day. I tried to concentrate and think. Did I sort all the mail, do the mis-sorts and send the reports? I had already made the necessary call and arranged for my relief to cover the office in case the doctor was running behind schedule.

My eyes scanned the room. The office itself was very large with lots of widows, the floor was lopsided, I had tested it myself with a small ball one boring afternoon. The ball automatically rolled from my starting place and landed on the other side of the room. The old plaster was falling from the ceiling and each day I swept up different areas of falling remnants as part of my duties. The building itself was a historical landmark. The residents of the small town of Clayson, had taken care that very few changes had been made to the building over the years. Only the major necessities, such as a bathroom with plumbing, (the old outhouse was still there) running water, and a real furnace had been installed.

The building was now called the Clayson Post Office where many long and boring days were spent as the newly appointed Postmaster. Hours would go by without seeing a single person. So most of my time was spent straightening up the files, recounting the stamp stock and talking on the phone. This morning dragged more than usual. No customers, no phone calls and very little mail to sort. There was nothing left to do but sit and wait out the slow-moving minutes.

Having been born and raised in this little town, the elementary school I attended when I was a child, was only a quarter of a mile up the road from where I was sitting. Clayson, RI. was my home, and I had lived there all my life. I was almost 54 now, divorced with three grown children, seven grandchildren and a great-grandchild on the way. I was so sure that my life would improve after the divorce. The promotion to Postmaster was what I had worked so hard for. I was determined to show everyone, especially myself, that I could become someone important. The struggle was definitely not worth it. Disappointment seemed to be my only friend. It was only a title. There was no substance behind it. Here I was in a run down building alone. No co-workers, no real responsibility. Only long and dreary days. My health had been deteriorating rapidly, and I kept telling myself that it was just the stress and that caused my depression. I almost had myself convinced, then the pain kept reminding me that it was not in my head but in my body.

That morning passed, and it was time to close up the building for lunch. I had to close the building down every day for two hours. Today I must leave quickly and get on my way to the doctors. I pulled the security shade down and locked the inside office door. The front door always remained open for any of the local residents to come in and retrieve their po box mail at their own leisure.

The drive to the doctor's office only took a short time and when I walked in, I was the only patient in the reception area.

The receptionist, Lotty, greeted me with a smile and brought me down the hall and did the usual weighing in. "My, Pam, you have lost a little weight. (My weight seldom fluctuates more than a pound or two). One Hundred and ten pounds, 5 foot 5 inches tall. You lost about 8 pounds, Pam. Is there anything unusual going on with you?"

Now I know that most women would be envious, but I had always wanted to be a little heavier with more curves. But a skinny little girl I had been as a child and now I am still a skinny woman.

Lotty looked at me and asked again, "Any special problem that brings you here today?"

"Oh just the usual change of life things, I think. But I want Dr. Jackie to check me out. I just don't feel comfortable with a male doctor at this point t in my life."

"Oh no problem, just get undressed and put the dressing gown on. Dr. Jackie will be in to see you shortly," Lottie stated with her usual smile.

It seemed like an eternity had passed until Jackie came back in the room. Jackie is a tiny woman, in her middle thirties. She was a pretty, with a lovely smile. "Well, it's nice to see you Pam," she said in her soft voice. "What can I help you with?"

I paused and gathered my strength and said, "I think I need to have you check me, probably a pap smear, as I have been having a great deal of spotting and have been experiencing great pain."

She smiled and said, "Well then, let me see what I can see."

I leaned back on the exam table and closed my eyes. I knew or at least I had a good idea of what was coming. Did you ever ignore that little voice in the back of your head? It doesn't lie, you know. Deep down inside of me I knew I was putting off the inevitable. Bad news.

Dr. Jackie got her array of instruments out and reached for the wonderful metal pap smear gadget, all of us women are familiar with, "The Spectrum."

I asked quietly, "Jackie, could you use something small as I have not had sex in almost five years, what with my divorce and everything?" She smiled and pulled up her little stool in front of the table and began the exam. In about ten seconds, I saw her face go white. She pulled back from the exam table and began to reach for cotton towels and paper towels. For those few seconds I had no idea what was going on. It wasn't until I felt the dampness between my legs that I knew I was bleeding. Bleeding doesn't quite describe what was happening, I believe that hemorrhaging is the correct word. She told me to remain still and she would return in a second.

"An ambulance is on the way, Pam. I have called your daughter and she will meet you at the hospital (R.I. Woman's Center). I have also called for some specialists to meet you there to examine you," Dr. Jackie replied.

Suddenly, my world had gone berserk. "What was going on, what did you see Jackie?"

"I am no expert in this area Pam, but I know that it is serious and that you must take care of this immediately. I want no argument, just get into the ambulance and go to the hospital. I will be in contact with the specialist, Dr. Johnson, as soon as we find out what is going on," Dr. Jackie replied.

I sat there on the table in shock. Shaking and terrified. Now what? I can't remember being more afraid. I tried to keep myself from crying. I knew it was bad, but never let myself think of a serious illness. Not me, this can't be. Not Pam. I am as healthy as a horse. I've never had any serious health problems. This is all just a bad dream.

A few minutes passed and in walked the ambulance drivers. They tried to be very gentle and assisted me in getting on the Gurney. Living in Clayson is as rural as one can get, even for the state of Rhode Island. It was very close to the Conn. state line, and most of the residents were either farmers or people who just wanted to get as far away from the city as possible. The hospital was a 20 minute drive. The EMT's asked all usual medical history questions and tried to keep me calm with conversation. (Everyone knows everyone else in a small town.) A few short minutes passed, and I was strapped in tightly and we were on our way. I knew then, that my world would soon change drastically.

The drive to the hospital went quickly. We arrived at the emergency entrance within fifteen minutes. The back doors opened and I saw my daughter Robin standing there with a cigarette in her hand. Her face looked as pale as I have ever seen it. Robin is a beautiful woman. She is 5'10" tall with long auburn hair. Her figure is like that of a model. Her eye's are a dark brown color and her complection is olive. I am not just speaking as a proud mother here, all one has to do is walk beside her and see the heads turn. It's not only the men that stare, but women as well. No one would ever guess that she has four children. Her type of beauty is rare. I have always thought of her as exotic looking.

Robin immediately ran toward the ambulance. "What's going on Mom? What's happening? Are you all right?"

Rah, (my nickname for her) I wish I knew. One minute I was being examined, and the next Dr. Jackie had me in the ambulance. I confessed to Rah, I am so glad to see you, I'm really nervous, and Dr. Jackie told me that she called you and she has also called some specialists that are supposed to meet me here."

The EMT's began pushing me on the Gurney toward the entrance door, Rah reached for my hand. I have not seen that look or felt that grip since she was a little girl. At that moment, she was my little girl once again.

Chapter 2
Examination

In the next 45 minutes all that Rah and I could do was wait. I had answered all the admission questions and filled out all the proper forms. I was then asked to sign a form called "A Living Will." Boy that was just what I needed. Nothing like reminding you that you might die. Rah stayed right next to me and only released my hand when it was necessary for me to sign papers. She was beginning to get angry. "Where is the Doctor? Why is no one looking at you? You could bleed to death." It was moments like this when Rah proved she was a really red head. Her temper was beginning to flare, and I tried to calm her down, and asked her to be patient.

"I am all right Rah. The bleeding has slowed down. Please stay calm for my sake."

The emergency doors were constantly swinging. It seemed as if there was not a moment when someone was either walking in or walking out. But thought all the congestion, I heard a familiar voice. It was my mother. Beside her were my youngest son Brandon and his wife Susan. My mother is your typical mom. Since she became a senior citizen, her attitude has become different. She still is an attractive woman, although the signs of age are beginning to show. But she is almost 80. Strong willed and thick headed, but with a soft heart. The problem is she keeps it locked so no one gets in. Not even as a child could, I penetrate it. I knew she loved me, but I just wish she could have told me more that she did. I needed to hear the words. But that was then, she was here now, and I was very happy to see her.

I looked at my son. Tears were in his eyes, and he appeared to be terrified.

My first instinct was to jump off the Gurney and hug him, but instead, I just smiled and said. "Hey Sonny Boy, I am glad you're here. I've gone and done it this time."

"Mom, what's wrong with you? What is happening?"

"I am not sure yet, I haven't seen any of the Doctors yet, but I had some hemorrhaging. So, Dr. Jackie sent me here," I replied.

"Why are you still in the hall? This is ridiculous! Where is the doctor?" Rah asked.

"I am sure that someone will see me soon. Can everyone just calm down? I am okay. Please!" I asked.

It was only a few short moments that passed, when a nurse in a brightly colored uniform came out of the examination area and smiled and said, "Your turn now Mrs. Ayers."

She started pushing the Gurney when Rah interrupted her and asked, "Can I go too, please?"

"That is no problem, just follow me." We went into exam room #three. Good, I thought, at least it is a good number.

"You will have to get undressed now, Mrs. Ayers," the nurse replied.

She left the room, and I started to undress. It was at that moment that Rah started crying. "Oh Mom, I am so sorry. I am trying to keep myself together, really. I am."

I held her in my arms and simply said, "I love you, and everything will be all right. We have to have some faith." I returned to the exam table and reclined, trying to prepare myself for what was coming. During this whole time, Rah held my hand.

In about five minutes two very young doctors came into the room. Honestly, they could have been my sons. They looked like young kids. All I could think of was, *oh please let me just cover myself up with the clean white sheet and become completely invisible.*

After a brief explanation regarding the disaster at Dr. Jackie's office, the little "stool" was properly placed, once again, in front of me. "Try and relax, Mrs. Ayers, I won't hurt you."

"I just need to take a quick look."

I closed my eyes and began to pray. It was the same prayer that I had been saying for almost a year. "Please give me the strength to face what is coming." Then a Hail Mary followed by The Lords Prayer. I opened my eyes to see a very interested look on the doctors puzzled face (or interns). I was never exactly sure who he was. He gave the other doctor permission to take a look.

I felt like an object on display. A very interesting and very sick object. They did not say anything to each other but quickly excused themselves with the promise that they would return shortly. I held another tight grip on my daughter's hand, and then breathed a sigh of relief. At least they didn't hurt me.

The next group of doctors arrived within a half an hour. The lead doctor was older, tall and very confident in his manners. He was accompanied by three other doctors (interns, or students). But this time, I could read what was on his name emblem. The word Oncology jumped out at me. I am no college graduate but that one word said it all.

He apologized for any discomfort I had, but asked permission to "take a look." I really didn't even answer him, I just laid back down on the table. It didn't take long, just a glance, and it was over. "Mrs. Ayers, I am going to admit you immediately. We need to do more tests. But what I see right now is a large tumor in your vagina."

Tumor? Tumor, did he just say a tumor? Oncologist? I knew then and there without any further testing required what was coming next. Suddenly, my hand felt like it was in a vice grip. Apparently Rah had put it all together as well.

"No, I can't today, Dr. Johnson. That's impossible and out of the question. I can return tomorrow morning and be admitted, if that is acceptable?" There were too many loose ends that had to be handled. Mostly Post Office problems, but arrangements had to be made.

The doctor frowned and said, "Well this is your life we are talking about, Mrs. Ayers. But tomorrow is okay as long as you are admitted by 9:00 a.m."

"I'll be here Doctor." He shook my hand and left with all the other doctors following him, acting like they were playing the game "Follow the leader." I got up from the examination table and without a word, began to get dressed. Rah started to say something, but I stopped her, and just quietly said, "not now Rah." I picked up my pocketbook from the floor and grabbed my coat. "Lets go" and we walked out of the door. The family was seated in the waiting room in a nice little circle. They stood up immediately upon seeing me. Before anyone could ask, I informed them of the finding of the tumor and that I had to return tomorrow for more tests and a biopsy.

"Oh my God, what do you mean a biopsy? Is it cancer? What did they say?" My mother asked.

"Mom, we will know more tomorrow. Can we just go home right now?" I quietly asked.

My mother's eyes were filled with tears and fear. She put her arms around me and began to cry. I can tell you the exact minute of when she had hugged me last. It was after the birth of my last child, Brandon. That was 30 years ago. That was just her way.

My son and daughter-in-law Susan were speechless. Brandon just sat down in a chair very quickly as if his legs had given out. I could see the grip he had on the arm of the chair. My eyes met his for only a second, and I smiled at him. God I loved him. He was my baby and had always been a good son. Why hadn't I told my children that I loved them more? Like Mother, like Daughter? I guess that's the way it works sometimes no matter how hard you try and change it.

"Lets go now, please?" I requested. Without any further words we left the area and walked through the automatic doors. I rode with Rah, and my mother rode with Brandon and Susan. I decided to stop at my house first, to get the information needed to inform my superiors about my illness. I reached down to get a tissue out of my pocketbook and noticed my socks. I had worn my most God awful socks to work this day. They were ugly red wool Christmas socks (in October). The Post office had been so damp and cold the past few days that I had needed something warm for my feet. *Well if that isn't a pretty picture?* I thought. I began to giggle.

"Mom, what are you laughing at?"

"Oh Rah, look at my socks. Can you imagine what the doctors must have thought?" Right then we both burst into laughter. It was wonderful to laugh!

There was no sleep for me that night; medications did not help as my mind was in a nonstop mode. The pain was getting bad again. Not quite time for another pill, I will just have to wait. I was so scared. I felt so alone. For that moment, I actually wished my ex-husband was with me to comfort me. It wasn't that I loved him anymore, the love had just evaporated. But I wouldn't have to be brave with him. He knew all my weakness and accepted them. Of course he had to constantly remind me about them. But the rest of the family thought I was a rock. If they only knew just how timid and frightened me was of what was coming,

Cervical Cancer. There I said it! I know that is what I have. I had not gotten a Pap Smear in years. But I had never had any problems with my periods or anything else. I never had cramps and except for the occasional spotting (in the past year) there were no signs of any problems. I just hope that it hasn't spread anywhere else. There was no history of cancer in my family. " I don't know why this has happened, but I do intend to find out," I said out loud. "I wish I had a medical book so I could look this up, but I will find out more tomorrow." I finally leaned back on the couch and closed my eyes. I was so very tired.

Chapter 3
Loose Ends

Daybreak finally came and I was already showered, dressed and ready to go. Rah had thrown a few things in a suitcase at some point in all the confusion of me in the hospital. I hoped she had not forgotten anything important. I could hear my mom and dad moving around quietly and whispering. They were afraid I might hear their conversation. They are too old to be facing this, I thought. God had blessed me with wonderful parents, and at that moment, I thanked him. Just like everyone else, I took things for granted. But not anymore. I promised myself that last night. I must remember to be thankful for everything that was given to me these past years. I am truly ashamed for not being thankful for all the blessings that had been given to me.

"Good morning Mom and dad!" I said.

"My mother's first question of the day was, "How did you sleep?"

"Not bad," I lied.

"I am all set and ready to go. I just want to get going." I had been creative and spent my early morning hours trying to make myself to appear more like "Pam." Especially after spending ten minutes crying while I was showering. Yes, I know that I am vain, and I will probably always be. But I will be damned if I am going down without a fight. Sick or not. Upon completion of my hair and makeup, I stood in front of the mirror and smirked. Yes, I did a very good job of disguising myself. I looked a little frail and the circles under my eyes were still visible, but unless you really knew me, you would think I looked pretty healthily. My illusion of a healthy, happy person was successful. No one could guess that my eyes had been filled with tears, and my heart was breaking an hour before. This was important to me as I had to go into the main post office and I did not want anyone to suspect anything regarding my failing health. I had worked in Providence for over a year on a detail and knew just about everyone. The rumors will fly anyway as soon as the news hits. That is just the way it is. But for now, I only wanted the major higher-ups to know of my illness.

"Do you want something to eat?" my mother asked.

"I don't think I should Mom, but I will have some coffee." My dad, who had been totally quiet since we arrived there last night, was sitting in his usual place at the table. I looked at him and saw a gentle man, tall and very thin. He was my step dad but very few. People even knew it. I admired him and loved him. He married my mom when I was nine years old. I never knew any father except him.

"How are you doing? Are you in pain Pam?" he asked calmly.

"Not too bad Dad. I'm actually doing pretty well, (lying again). I just want to get this over with. I already know what's wrong with me."

"Perhaps you shouldn't be so sure, your no doctor," dad advised. Give them a chance, Pam. It's going to be okay. I have confidence in you. You're a strong woman."

The nerve pill and pain medication had begun to take effect again. I was feeling a bit more relaxed. Now all I had to do was wait for Rah to arrive. I had three hours to get to the hospital and to the Post office. "Plenty of time," I said out loud.

My dad looked at me, "What did you say?'

"Oh I was just thinking out loud dad. I think it is the medication making me a little stranger than I normally am." He smiled and continued reading the paper.

Just then my mom came back into the kitchen. She was now dressed and ready to go. "Where is Robin? She should be here," she asked, concerned.

"Not to worry mom, she'll be here. She has to get the kids ready and off to school, and that is no easy accomplishment." Within fifteen minutes the door bell rang. It was Rah. I went to the door and let her in. "We're all set, everything okay with the kids?"

"Yea, I've got it handled Mom. Don't worry."

"Okay, lets go before I lose my courage." So we were off and running with my suitcase in hand.

Everyone was very quiet as we headed toward Providence. I was concerned about my mom. She had already had two heart attacks, and I know that this ordeal was not going to do her heart any favors. I tried to keep the conversation on the lighter side, with small talk. No mention of my illness allowed. We mostly discussed Rah' children and the usual morning confusion in getting them ready for school. To my knowledge, the kids were told nothing about their "Meme's illness." I earned that little nickname from the first grandchild, Amanda. She could not say the French name for gramma which is Mim May, so lucky me, Meme stuck.

We pulled in the parking lot of the main post office and I asked Rah and my mother to stay put in the car. "They won't let you in anyway. Besides, I'll only be a minute or two." With some effort I got out of the car. Once inside the building I could see the usual line of people standing waiting to make their purchases. Walter, a tall, thin, black man was standing in front of the two elevators. His job was to monitor the coming and going of all visitors. He would check and make sure that you had an ID badge before you were allowed in the elevator. "Going Postal" had been in the news recently so careful attention was being paid to exactly who was entering the building.

Walter is a pleasant man and immediately recognized me. "Well hello Pam! I haven't seen you in a long time. How are you?

"Oh I'm fine Walter. My little office has been keeping me very busy. How are you?" I asked.

"Just as fit as ever," he said, with a big smile on his face. The elevator door open and I hurried in.

"Talk to you later." The door closed and all I could think was "Going Up" and pushed the third floor button. I hope I don't see anyone that I know before I get into Mr. Wilsons office. The doors opened. One large inhale and I stepped out into the corridor. *Secretly, I wished then that I had taken another nerve pill before I had left. One pill is good, two is better. (At least that is what they say) Too late now, Here I go.*

Mr. Wilson's secretary, Marla, was sitting at her desk talking on the phone. She glanced up and gave me a nod and a smile. She was an attractive woman with a reputation of being a top notch secretary. She pointed to a chair and smiled again. *Oh good*, I thought. *She hasn't heard anything about me yet.* I could tell by her mannerisms that no rumors had reached her as yet. I quickly sat down in the direction she had pointed to and looked around. The office was nicely decorated with the usual plants and paintings. All very fitting for the man with the title of Postmaster of Rhode Island.

Marla finished her conversation and quickly announced me to Mr. Wilson. Before she could ask me any questions, Mr. Wilson came out of his office. His looks fit his title. He was an older man with a balding head and slightly over weight. He came toward me with his hand held out. "Pam please come into my office."

"I can only stay a few minutes. I have another an appointment in just a short amount of time," I stated. We entered his office and he held the chair for me. "I have to be in the hospital for further tests, Mr. Wilson."

"What can I do? You name it Pam. Take all the time you need. Arrangements have already been made for your office to be covered. I don't want you to worry about anything. Just get yourself better," he said sincerely.

"I can't thank you enough for you kindness. I will do the best that I possibly can. Thank you again. I really have to leave now. Good bye, Mr. Wilson, I will keep you posted." He shook my hand and walked me out of the room.

I walked out of his office and just nodded my head at his secretary. I just had to leave and leave quickly. It was Mr. Wilson who had given me my promotion as Postmaster. Tears were filling my eyes, and my throat had a huge lump in it. The elevator seemed as if it was a hundred miles away. I kept my eyes down and just kept walking. Thank God I met no one that I had known. When I finally reached the elevator it seemed like an hour passed until the doors opened and I stepped in. "Going down." When the doors opened again, Walter was no where to be seen. I hurried out the front doors. I had made it, no one saw me, no questions to answer, and no fake smiles on my face.

I reached the car as fast as I could. The intense pain was returning and movement was getting extremely difficult. I could see my mom was crying when I got to the car. Rah was talking to my mother, and I could only imagine what was being said. When I opened the door, I startled them. They were so busy in conversation that they did not see me coming. "Would you please drive Rah?" "I don't think that I am physically able to drive right now."

"Okay mom, just get in and I will get you to the hospital as fast as I can." Thanks to her fast driving we reached the hospital in record time.

"Take me to the emergency entrance. You can park the car in the lot and meet me at the emergency doors. The less I had to walk the better." It's hard to hide the pain from people you love sometimes. Be brave Pam and smile.

Chapter 4
Admissions

I leaned against the wall next to the door and waited. The receptionist saw me standing there and asked, "Can I help you?"

"Yes, I am just waiting for my daughter. I will be right there. I am scheduled to be admitted this morning."

"May I have your name, please?"

"Pamela Ayer," I replied softly.

Rah and my mom came through the doors just at that moment, and joined me at the wall. The admission went smoothly. All my paperwork was ready and I had been assigned a room. Room # 411 (another good number, this has to be a sign) The nurse came out of the exam room with a wheel chair and asked me to sit. Which I did without any argument. She chatted briefly with Rah all the time heading me toward the elevators. I was in so much pain by then, I felt like the breath was being squeezed out of me. We reached the fourth floor and quickly entered my room. The smell of disinfectant was really strong. I could feel my stomach start to turn.

"I feel really sick to my stomach. I need to go to the bathroom." I reached for the bars on the wall next to the toilet. I was vomiting everything I had put in my stomach that morning. I could hear the voices in the next room. I knew that they could hear me as well. I splashed water on my face and held onto the sink taking a few deep breaths. "I can do this. I can do this." I opened the door and walked out into my new little home trying to smile. The nurse was still talking to Rah and my mom when I exited the bathroom.

"How are you feeling, Mrs. Ayer? I can get you something for your stomach if you wish?" the nurse asked.

"Oh, I feel a little better now, the medication and my nerves just didn't mix."

"Well, if you need anything, the Nurses call button is on the right arm on the bed. The doctor should be in to see you very soon. "He is doing his rounds right now, and will see you before he has to return to his office."

"Okay, but before you leave, is it okay for me to have something to drink, like a cup of coffee?" I asked.

"No coffee," she was fast to advise. But I will have something sent up from the cafeteria in a few minutes. You can drink water. I know that won't interfere with your tests."

Rah started to organize the clothes from my suitcase and my personal items. "Mom, you didn't bring anything to read. I'll go down to the gift shop, if you like, and get you some magazines? And while I am down on the first floor, I will check on getting you a phone."

"Let's hope that I am not here long enough to need the phone. But it is a good idea, thanks Rah."

While we were alone, my mother came over to the bed and said, "Just how long have you known about this? Why didn't you have this checked sooner?"

"Mom, I was checked by three different doctors. They all were concentrating on my stomach, and they all came up with the same diagnosis. It's your nerve. You're under a lot of pressure. All three of them thought it was depression and prescribed antidepressants and sedatives. And with what was happening in my life. I agreed with them. Besides, I had all the symptoms of going through the change of life as well. So the diagnosis seemed right on the money. Life hasn't been to peachy for me lately Mom. I am losing my beautiful home. You know that I can't sell it. My ex really screwed me on that. But I don't want to think or talk about it right now. The only good thing about this tumor is that it kept my mind off money problems." Mom continued to scold me, but at that point, I was not listening to what she was saying. I really didn't need to hear this right now.

"Pam, Pam, are you listening to me? Are you all right?" she asked.

"Mom, I am just about scared out of my mind. I am just really petrified. Can we change the subject for a little while?" Just then a voice came through the speaker over my head. It was the nurse. "Mrs. Ayer, I am sorry but you cannot have any solid foods until later. Only clear liquids for now. If you need anything, just push the button."

"Okay, I said. Not only are they going to torture me, they are planning on starving me as well. Great! Now what? I'll just lose a few more pounds. What's the difference at this point?" I said feeling pitiful.

"You shouldn't have a bad attitude Pam. They will treat you better if you are nice. Listen and do what I tell you to do. I am still your mother."

"Mom, I don't feel like being little misses nice patient. All my life that is what I have been. Nice and polite, never say the wrong thing to anyone. That is why I lived in such a disastrous marriage for so long. I really believed that I should be the perfect wife and the perfect mother. A lot of good it did me. Look at me now!"

Rah walked in the door with a handful of magazines and newspapers. It was good timing on her part, as I was getting very upset with my mom. I did not want that to happen.

"Here you go, Mom. Hope this will keep you busy enough."

"I just hope they leave me alone long enough so that I get the chance to read them. I think that I should go and put the dressing gown on, before the nurse or the doctor comes in. Excuse me for a few minutes." Getting myself undressed proved to be quite difficult and painful. In addition the result was totally unattractive. Little blue diamonds were going to be the patterns for today's outfit. "*Gosh, this is becoming,* I thought. *It just complements my skinny figure totally.*

My Mom was sitting in the chair by the window crying, and Rah was attempting to get the television to work when I made my fashion entrance. Totally lovely, was the comment from Rah.

"You like? I thought you might. I must remember to bring this home with me."

"Mom, your phone works, I just checked it."

"Great, I might need to make my escape fast. It's comforting to know that I can reach you in a hurry."

"I'll be here faster than a bullet, all you have to do is call," Rah said smiling.

" Time for me to get back in the bed, and permission or no permission, I am taking a pain pill." I slid my way back into bed. God I was tired. I tried to position my self so that I would feel a little better. "Rah, please get me a pain pill from my pocketbook and a glass of water."

"Right away Mom," she said and moved quickly toward my purse.

Chapter 5
Visitors

A short time after taking the medication I could hear footsteps on the tile floor, coming in my direction. I started to get nervous, thinking it must be the doctor and his "Team." Instead, to my pleasant surprise in walked Brandon and Susan. Right behind them was my older son Jason and his wife Ann. Susan leaned over and kissed me with tears in her eyes. To my surprise, the others did the same thing. They stood waiting their turn and then kissing me gently. I was just about to say something, when the phone rang. I just about jumped out of my skin, it startled me so. I reached for the receiver and said "Hello?"

"Pam it's me. What the heck is going on? Brandon said you have Cancer. Is it true?" I was so surprised to hear his voice. I couldn't say a word. It had been almost two ½ years since I had spoken to my ex. I was at a total loss for words.

I paused for a minute and then said, "I don't know for sure yet, they will do a biopsy sometime today."

"Are the children there with you?"

"Yes, all of them are here with me."

"I call you back later," he said. "Click," I heard the phone go dead.

I hung up and I guess the tone of the conversation or the look on my face said it all. "Who was that?" Rah asked.

"That was your father" The room went silent.

"Great," was all that Rah verbalized. The disgusted look on her face was mirrored by everyone else in the room. My ex had earned that reaction from

24

his children, but I won't think about that now. I will just think about it tomorrow. That's my favorite saying. God Bless "Scarlet."

The gathering in the hospital room reminded me of a family reunion. Christmas time or birthday parties were about the only occasions when my three children were all in the room at the same time. Typically one would be upset with the other one for some stupid reason. I looked at them all. I had such a beautiful family. My daughter is beautiful, and my son's are handsome. At that moment, my heart was so filled with pride, but at the same time, my body was being invaded by cancer.

When was the last time I was kissed by my sons, I can't remember? But right this minute they were all here. It was a dose of good medicine for me. I was not about to leave my children. No, not yet.

The nurse came in the room and immediately showed her disapproval. "There are too many people in here. "Some of you will have to leave."

"Well, we just got here," Jason spoke up.

"Perhaps a few of you could go down to the cafeteria and get some coffee?"

"I'll go, Rah said. I need a cigarette anyway."

"Boy, I could sure use one myself," I said smiling.

"I can get you a patch, if that would help?" suggested the nurse.

"Thank you, and I would appreciate it very much." I took a pain pill a few minutes ago, nurse. I was just too uncomfortable."

"Well, someone will be in to take a blood test, what type of pain medication did you take?"

"Eight hundred milligrams of something. I can't remember the name. They gave me the prescription when I was in the emergency room yesterday."

The nurse just nodded and said, "I will make a note of it on your chart and find out what pain medication it was."

"How long are you going to be in here?" Asked Susan.

"I have no idea. They really haven't told me anything yet."

Jason finally broke his silence. "Well where is the doctor, I want to talk to him.

"Jay, I am sure he will be here shortly.

"Mom, why didn't you tell someone you were sick?"

"I explained it to your Grandmother. I did see a doctor. I saw three different ones. They all thought it was just stress and depression."

"Well, if you ask me, I think it's all Dad's fault. If you didn't have so many worries, you wouldn't have gotten sick," Jay replied.

25

"Please Jay, lets not go there right now, okay?"

His wife Ann came over and sat on the bed. She took my hand and asked, "Is there anything you need?" She is such a sweet woman. She was not at all what I pictured that Jay would marry. Jay had always been very particular on the appearance of the women he dated. All of them gorgeous. And then wham, he brings home Ann and before I knew it, they were married. Ann was slender, tall and very thin. She has a pretty face, but never wears any makeup. She never bothers with her hair and it's such a pretty color. It's what you would call strawberry blonde. But she loves Jay. And he is not easy to live with. That I am sure of. Jay is very much like his father. He would deny that with every emotion he has, but it is a true statement. He is very stubborn and thickheaded. But he is a wonderful father. That was not one of his father's traits. Brandon is a good dad as well. I think they both tried extra hard to be what their father wasn't. They both are good husbands. At least I think they are. Neither one of my sons either drinks or cheats. They spend all their spare time with their wives and daughters. Not so with their father. He drank and was always out shooting pool or something. Sometimes not coming home until four in the morning. But he always had a hell of a story. An unbelievable one, but he always made sure he had an excuse.

The only time my ex spent with his children was when it was doing something he liked to do. Such as fishing or hunting. I believe that his sons love him. But I think it is because they know that it is what is expected of them. I know that there is no real bond between them. They avoid their father like a bill collector. Occasionally, he can catch them on the phone. But they never go to visit their dad, not even on his birthday or Christmas unless they are totally trapped into it. Why should they? He never remembers their birthdays or their children's birthdays. God please forgive me for loving a man that selfish.

Two years before the divorce, my ex was diagnosed with being Bipolar with Paranoid Schizophrenia. Here I go thinking about the past again. I have got to stop thinking about it. I can feel another panic attack approaching. "Mom, would you please get me my pocketbook."

"I definitely need another anxiety pill." Always the same reaction in my body when talking about my ex. These little pink pills had been the only medicine that I had found which actually worked in controlling these attacks.

My ex had spent almost three weeks in the Mental Health hospital. It all started when OJ Simpson was arrested for the alleged murder of his wife. I remember it exactly. My ex started staying up all night and watching tv. When I questioned him on it, he began to tell me that the tv was talking to him, and that I could not use the phone. Now one must realize that this came right out of the blue. There were no noticeable signs of this earlier. Of course my ex had always been controlling, but he was a Correctional Officer. I thought, the personality fit the position. But his actions became really weird. He even went as far as to go to the State Police barracks and report to them that an alien had taken over my body. Luckily one of the state troopers had worked with him at the prison and knew that something was terribly wrong. He called the Post Office and told me of the situation and I drove where they were holding him. The trooper informed me how to get in contact with the prison employee counselors and try to get some help for him. I tried everything that was in my power and so did the counselors, but to no avail. You cannot admit your spouse to an institution unless he is dangerous to himself or someone else. They have to sign themselves in. Needless to say, that was not going to happen. As far as he was concerned, it was I that was not normal. So, as it turned out, one night he took a ride with the dog to Canada. He packed nothing. He had no idea where he was going. I had spent many nights without any sleep because I was afraid that he was going to kill me. But that night I was just too exhausted to stay awake. When I awoke in the morning, he was gone. I put out a missing persons' report and waited. Three days passed, and I received a call from a city in upstate NY. He had been arrested. Apparently, he had frightened some receptionist in a hotel and was talking crazily. She called the police, and he was soon placed in their mental hospital. So the rest is history. His sons went after him and brought him home. Upon his arrival back in RI he signed himself in our mental hospital. He spent about three weeks in the locked unit. I remember that I had to go through four locked doors just to visit him. I visited him every day, leaving work early so that I could be with him. And when I tell you I was scared to death every time I went through those doors, it is no exaggeration.

This is when the doctors informed me that he was Bipolar with Paranoia and was also a schizophrenic. They suggested shock treatments for him, but I refused. They put him on all kinds of medication, which did work and he came home. There's more, much more, but I have had enough thoughts about him. It's time for me to start focusing on myself and my health.

Chapter 6
The Tests Begin

In came a young pretty nurse pushing a small cart with equipment on it. "Good morning everyone. "I just have to take some blood and I will be right out of here." She placed a rubber tourniquet around my forearm and quickly took two vials of blood. She smiled and said, "there that didn't hurt, did it? By for now, but I'll be back." And she was gone.

"Gee, I hope the rest of the tests are that easy," I said with a sigh of relief.

It wasn't long after that, and the doctor walked into the room. He had his usual "Team" with him. I got a much better look at him this morning. He was very nice looking and extremely confident in himself. "Good morning, Mrs. Ayer. I have you scheduled for quite a few tests today. The biopsy will take place early tomorrow after I have had a chance to study all your tests from today."

"Well, what are we looking for Doctor?"

"I won't smooth anything over. I am already sure that we are dealing with Cervical Cancer. It appears the tumor grew downward in your vagina, which could be to your advantage." I am considering a complete hysterectomy, just to be on the safe side, but as I said, I want to wait for the results of to days' test before that decision is made. Today you are scheduled for chest x-rays, a cat scan, and a blood oxygen test. In addition of course the biopsy tomorrow. "Do you have any questions?"

Questions, is he kidding? Where do I start? I thought. "I am not sure what to ask?" I answered.

"Why don't we wait until tomorrow? The picture will be much clearer then. I will be changing your pain medication. Just something a little stronger, as I know that you must be very uncomfortable. Your family can stay if they wish, but you won't be in your room very much once the tests get started." He turned at looked at my family and said, "You can call my office if you have any questions. I will get back to you as soon as possible. Well that's about it for now, Mrs. Ayer. I won't be giving you any exam right now as I do not wish to disturb the tumor at this time. I will see you again later on this afternoon. Goodbye for now," and he turned and left with his "Team" right behind him.

My mind was spinning. How am I going to handle all of this? If I don't work, I don't get paid. The post office does not take Temporary Disability Insurance out of your pay. "Oh God, more money worries." It would probably be better to let the cancer just take me. I don't think I want to care anymore. I am so sick and so depressed about everything I don't know if I can handle it. "Scarlett O'Hara," I'll just think about Scarlett.

I looked around the room and saw the look of devastation on my family. Susan turned away from me, but I saw the tears rolling down her face. One by one they all turned away and looked at each other. I knew they were all scared. They were all trying to conceal their fears from me.

Rah was the first one to speak. "Does anyone want to go for coffee with me?" Her voice was shaking.

"I'll go," said Brandon.

"Me too," replied his wife Susan.

"Rah, will you bring me so tea and maybe some crackers?" "My mouth tastes terrible."

"Maybe the crackers will help my stomach."

"We'll be right back," and they left the room.

I asked my mom, 'How did you like the doctor? "

"He seemed nice, but who were all those people with him?"

"Those are his associates. " "He is a Cancer Specialist."

"But just how does he know that you have cancer?" Her voice was getting very loud. When she gets nervous, her voice goes up a tone or two.

"Mom, you have to face the facts. I know the doctor is right. But I am not dead yet. We have to have faith. If Gram was here, she would say exactly those words to you. "Right now, let's remain calm and take the wait and see attitude."

At that moment I wished to myself that they would all go home, and let me face this alone. I get more upset looking at my family than thinking about the cancer. I wish I had enough courage to say it to them. But they wouldn't understand. They would only be hurt.

29

Chapter 7
Departure

Rah brought back my tea and crackers in about fifteen minutes. Long enough for a serious family discussion to have taken place in the cafeteria. Wish I could have been there. Rah, was the take charge type with her brothers. She was six years older than Brandon, but I know that Brandon had a great deal of respect for his sister. I have always realized that they were not close in the sense like some brothers and sisters, but I am sure that he would take any advice that Rah came up with. Jay and Rah were four years apart in age, and they seldom ever agreed on anything. But I am sure that Jay would take Rah's advise concerning me regarding the cancer.

Another nurse made her entrance. Only this one had a wheel chair. "Sorry everyone, but I have to take her down stairs for x-rays."

"You should all go home now I said to the group standing there. There is nothing that you can do. Why don't you call me later on this afternoon, and maybe some of you can come back later this evening?"

"Is that what you want, Mom?"

"Yes, I think that it would be best."

"Okay, come on everyone, lets go," Rah ordered.

"I'll call you later. Please, stop worrying all of you. I will be fine."

One by one they approached me, hugs and kisses and tears before they left the room.

"Nice family," the nurse said smiling.

"Thank you, I know. There all good kids, and my mom is the "typical mom"" in every sense of the word. No matter how old I get. She still orders me around."

The nurse smiled and said, "Well, it's time to go. Get in the chair, and we are on our way."

"Where is the x-ray department?" I asked.

"The bottom floor in the basement," she replied. She pushed me down the long corridor to the elevators. She tried to make small talk along the way to ease my nerves. But I was still scared to death, and I know that she could see it in my face.

Chapter 8
Tests

The basement was just that. A basement. It was one of the dreariest places I have ever seen. It had all the elements of a great horror movie. There were long fluorescence bulbs hanging from the ceilings. Some of the bulbs were blinking. Others were not working at all. The walls were painted dark grey with dull and dinghy grey tiles on the floor. We passed a few hospital employees as we moved along the corridor. They were talking and laughing, carrying their coffee to their destinations somewhere in the hospital.

Finally we arrived to the area where the above sign said x-ray Department. She pushed me into the room and there I sat waiting for the x-rays to take place. "Follow me, yet another nurse said, and I walked into the adjoining room. I was not placed on a table this time. I stood against the wall, and the large machine swung in front of me. I took a deep breath. *I thought, it's funny how the people who are taking the x-rays either stand or sit behind some protective wall or lead aprons. What's the matters, don't you want to get cancer? Bad girl Pam. Don't think that way. To them it is just a job, and I am positive they couldn't care less what your x-ray's results are. Why should they? Now just stand still and behave yourself, I thought. There were only a few more clicks of the machine to go, and I would be finished. One test down, just a few more to go.*

I was ushered into my wheel chair again, and pushed back to my room. When I got back to my room, it was just a little after twelve noon. Thank goodness, there is a tray with some food on it. I sat onto my bed and pulled the tray up carefully right in front of me. It had been a long time since I had some food in my stomach, what with losing it when I first arrived in the room. Now I felt famished. The food on the tray consisted of a beef bullion soup, Jello and clear tea. I was really surprised on how good it actually tasted. I reached for one of the magazines that Rah had purchased and tried to settle down and relax lying on the hospital bed.

About an hour passed, when a young man entered my room with a gentle knock on the door. "Mrs. Ayer?' I am here to take you to your Cat Scan."

"Oh, okay." I had never had a scan before, but I knew a few people who had and said they were easy to take. So I was not afraid. I climbed into the chair once again, and was off at the starting gate one more time. Same elevators, same lower floor. Definitely not one of my favorites, the lovely basement. Wouldn't you think with all the money that hospitals and doctors charge that the basement could be redone and look a little more cheerful? At least just a little bit? God bless some poor little child going down there for a test. They would be totally horrified.

As we left the elevator, all I could think of was a scarey Halloween movie I had seen. Some maniac was chasing his latest victim with his usual large knife in the basement of some hospital. Guess I have seen just too many horror movies. Anyone that knows me, knows that horror movies are my thing. I make sure I never watch any love stories or very few comedies. I escape to the world of either horror or science fiction. Lt. Ripley was my hero in the science fiction category. Of course Scarlett is always ever present in my mind. I read her story when I was in my early twenties. She was some woman. But back to reality. I do know the difference you know. But letting my mind wander is good for me and takes some of the fears away. At least for a few minutes.

The Cat Scan Department was a mirror image of the x-ray Department. But this time, I was helped onto a table. The room was dimly lighted with no windows. The employees were pleasant, and one young man explained the procedure to me, in step by step details. He was going to inject me with a dye (of some sort) and then take the pictures with the scan. Sounds easy enough. They only catch was, I might be allergic to the dye itself and have some form of reaction. But with any luck on my side, I would have no reaction and everything would go well. I was placed on the table with the machine whirring all around me. Lights flashed constantly, with the thoughts of my future spinning and flashing as well in my brain. *I wondered if any of these technicians had ever been in my position. Could they see my fear? Was I putting on a good face? My thoughts were getting harder to control. I tried with all my might to think of my grand children. Think positive Pam.*

33

But there was no light at the end of the tunnel, (no pun intended). Just dark roads ahead.

The machine was slowing down and so were the flashing lights. Oh good, it's over. I was feeling a little groggy and dizzy. Perhaps I was having a reaction to the dye. The technicians helped me back onto my little traveling bed. All I kept thinking was just take me back to my room. I want to go to sleep. I tried to stay awake on the return trip to the hospital room but everything was getting blurry.

I can just barely remember getting onto the bed and turning on my side when sleep finally came. I have no idea how long I slept. When I awoke, the first person I saw was my daughter Rah sitting by the window. In her hand was a bundle of crushed tissues. All that I could see was my poor little girl crying. She must have noticed me moving and quickly dropped the tissues in the waste basket next to her chair.

"Hi Rah. How long have you been here? Are you alone?"

"Yes Mom, I just couldn't stay away. They told me at the Nurses station that you had gone for your cat scan. Are you feeling okay?"

"Better now, I really needed some sleep. Also, I had something to eat. The food wasn't bad at all. I just hope the biopsy goes that easy. How is my Mom holding up?" I asked.

"She's not that great. You know how Nana can be. But Grampa really got on her case this afternoon. I really think she listened to him for a change."

"Good, I don't like to think of her getting herself all upset. We both can't be in the hospital at the same time. That would be a heck of a mess."

"I know, but I think that she is attempting to deal with it after Grampa said his piece."

"I hope so Rah, I said with a small smile. Are you going to be staying for a while Rah? I don't think they will be doing any more tests, at least not for a while."

"Don't worry Mom. I'll stay right here. I am not going to leave you" Amanda is at home with the kids and Greg will be home shortly. I think he will be coming in to see you after he feeds the kids and cleans up. I think he is going to bring Nana with him."

"That is nice of him, but he really doesn't have too. There is really nothing he can do. He wants to come, ma. I know he teases you a lot, but he really loves you."

"Greg and I have had our differences, but I believe he is a good man and a good father."

"Oh Mom, I love you. I am so scared. You can't leave me!"

"I have no intention of letting this cancer kill me. You know that I am tough and a fighter, so just don't worry. Everything is going to be all right. I can take just about anything, but a dentist."

"She laughed and said. "I know how much you like them."

"So you see Rah, this is going to be a slight detour in my life. I have to fight with every thing that I have got. Okay? I need you to be strong."

We spent the next few hours just enjoying each others company. We stayed away from the topic of illness and watched some tv and talked about the kids. Rah had four beautiful children. First was the one and only Amanda. She was sixteen and pregnant. Blonde and beautiful. Then came the lovely Tawnee (redhead), the comedian Haley (another red head) and last but by no means little Kyle. The one and only grandson. Brandon has two girls, Alex and Brianna and Jason has one girl, little Cheyenne. So you can see, I was never at a loss for company. I was the official babysitter, whenever I had the time. But I enjoyed it. I loved each and every one of those kids.

Unfortunately, our alone time was interrupted by a large round-faced nurse. She tapped on the door and walked in.

"Time for another test. I bet you thought we were through with you, didn't you? Well, I think this one might be a little uncomfortable for you."

"Well, okay, let's get it done." Rah came closer to me and held my hand.

"I just need to get a sample of your blood gases. I do have to go quite deep with the needle, but I will do it as fast as I can."

"Now I know that I have been saying how brave I am, but let me tell you this. This test was a pip. Hurt, oh my yes. I brought three children into the world and I don't think it hurt as badly as this little test." I squeezed Rah's hand until it turned white.

"Okay, I think I got enough blood for the test," the nurse said.

"Thank goodness that is over with," I admitted. The nurse smiled, took her little sample and said good bye. I relaxed back in the bed, studying my hand. You could see the black and blues beginning to show. In an hour or two, my whole hand will appear to be bruised.

"Rah, would you get me a cold cloth from the bathroom? Maybe that will help keep the bruising to a minimum and keep the swelling down?"

"Right away Mom."

I wrapped the cloth around my hand and closed my eyes. "That was no picnic," I commented. What was coming next?

35

Chapter 9
Passing Time

It was four o'clock when I opened my eyes. I had fallen asleep again. "Oh Rah, I am so sorry. I fell asleep again."

"It's good for you Mom. Just rest. I called Nana while you were sleeping and she is coming in with Greg tonight. I am not sure but I think Jay and Ann will be coming in also. But not Brandon and Susan. He wanted me to tell you that he would see you tomorrow. They couldn't get anyone to stay with the kids."

"They don't have to do this, there is nothing anyone can do but sit and look at me. Besides, I plan on being out of here tomorrow. I just have to get through this biopsy tomorrow morning. I only ask one thing from you Rah, that you be here when I wake up. I will feel better knowing that you are here. As silly as that sounds, I need you to be here."

"Mom, I wouldn't be anywhere else. Don't worry, I promise. I will be here waiting for you. I'll try and get here before you even go for the test in the morning. Do you know what time you are scheduled to have it?"

"No, I don't have a clue. Maybe someone at the Nurses station can tell you. If I don't see the doctor again and have the chance to ask him, would you check for me before you leave today?"

"Will do, so don't worry about it mom. I'll be here."

A young candy striper came in with a tray of food. "Oh good, is it real food or something just to keep me from being faint?

"Well, kind of just something to keep your strength up. After the tests. I am

36

sure you will get some solid foods."

The little candy striper was correct. Jello again and some soup. "Terrific," I commented. "I can feel my muscles getting stronger as I swallow this strawberry jello, Rah."

She laughed and said," just finish it ma, and no more teasing."

"The nurse gave me some new medication before you came Rah, it seems to be helping me, quite a bit."

"I'm glad mom, I hate to think of you being in pain. The rest of the family should be coming shortly. I wanted to ask you before they got here, did Dad ever call you back?"

"No he didn't, and if I was placing any bets on this, I would bet on that he never calls again." (I was 100% correct, he never called agin. Not once during the whole illness.

"Mom, he is one selfish man."

"Don't Rah, it doesn't do any good. Remember he is sick. You know that he is really not responsible for his actions. Try not to think bad thoughts. People like him pay later on, maybe not in this lifetime, but sometime. I believe that with my whole heart. I just keep telling my self, don't expect and you don't get disappointed. Remember that. He is not a happy man. "Think about it, would you want to be him even with all his money? He can't take it with him."

"That's for sure. Yea, but why you Mom, why not him?

"I believe that God has a plan for all of us. The good Lord did not point his finger at me and say "I shall make Pam sick. You can't blame God. It's just one of those things."

Greg arrived with my mom right on schedule. Neither of these two people were the best of friends under any circumstances. My mom had a tendency to dislike all of her own families mates. No one was ever good enough for us in her eyes. I think it was just the love she felt for us, she just wanted us to be happy. That was her way.

Greg had tried to overlook her opinions and was always pretty polite to her. The ride to the hospital must have been difficult for the both of them. "Hi Mom, Greg smiled and he came over to me and gave me a kiss.

"Hi Greggy Pooh." Don't ask where that little nickname came from, because I honestly don't know. I just started calling him that one day and it stuck.

Mom came over to the bed and sat down. "Now tell me every thing they did to you today. What is the matter with your hand? Did a nurse do that to you? Has your doctor been back in to see you yet?"

"No, the doctor hasn't been in again, and I am fine. My hand is just a little bruised from a blood test. I am fine. Rah was here with me when the test was taken. I've had some supper and I am feeling a little better. Just the biopsy is left. It's almost over and I will be home again.

"Well that is something that has to be discussed, she replied. You are not going to be going home alone," using her firmest tone of voice.

"Well we will discuss that later on Mom, when all this testing is over with. Okay mom?"

We all sat around and chatted about things in general. Rah and Greg were trying to find me a decent movie channel on the tv, but no luck. Of course there were no horror movies in the hospitals channel line up. I made a promise to myself, that when I got home that was the first thing I would watch. A good scarey movie.

The announcement came over the loud speaker that all visitors had to leave. Visiting hours were over with. Goodbyes were said with hugs and kisses and promises of returning visits tomorrow. And then they were gone and I was alone, at least for a little while.

Chapter 10
More Company

There was a knock on my door.

Not another test, I thought.

"Mrs Ayer?"

"Yes," I said.

"May I come in and speak with you for a moment?" she asked.

My door opened and in walked a woman whom I did not know. She was not a nurse or a doctor. She was a very attractive older woman. Very well groomed (department store type) and quite elegant looking with a lovely smile. Her hair was dark with streaks of grey placed in all the precise areas in her hair . Her make-up was perfect. "Hello Mrs. Ayer, my name is Ellen Pool. I am the Cancer Counselor for the hospital. I thought that I would just drop by and visit with you for a few moments if you are up to it.?"

"It's very nice to meet you. Is there something I can do for you?" I asked.

"Oh no, it's nothing like that, she said. I just wanted to let you know that I am available for counseling if you would like to talk someone. We have a special group that meets once a week, just to talk. We were hoping you would like to join us for a meeting when you are feeling up to it."

"Thank you for your kindness and the invitation, Mrs. Pool. I will let you know as soon as I get feeling a little better."

She leaned over and handed me her card. "You can call me anytime of the day or night. I'll let you get some rest. Please think it over, and call me Best of luck to you and may God be with you."

"Thank you again, and I know God is always with me," I replied.

I waited a few minutes until I was sure that there was going to be no more company and then I let myself cry. Not a little cry, but an alright hysterical, let the tears flow gusher. My tears came until there were none left to shed. I am not sure, but I think the tears helped. I don't know why Mrs. Pool's visit upset me so. Perhaps I am more tired than I realized.

I pushed the Nurses button, and requested a sleeping pill. I knew that especially tonight that there would be no sleep without chemical assistance. The nurse came in shortly and gave me he little white pill that I would define as a miracle worker. Sleep came very quickly.

Chapter 11
Biopsy

I opened my eyes to see a young Spanish girl standing next to my bed. "I am so sorry to wake you Mrs. Ayer, but I have to give you an unpleasant enema. It is a requirement for your surgery."

"What?" I was still half asleep. "Now? It's still dark outside. What time is it?"

"It is about 5:30 in the morning. The surgery you are to have is to begin at approximately 6:30 a.m."

"It is, Oh God." I was really hurting. I had not taken any pain medication before I fell asleep last night and I was paying for it now. My hand was still swollen and totally black and blue. "This was not going to be a good day." I won't even try to describe the discomfort I was in down in the lower area of my body, and just the thought of having an enema was about to kill me.

"I know," she said calmly. I'll be as fast and as gentle as I can be."

I explained to her that my tumor was pressing on my bowels and that she really needed to be careful. I don't know if she really cared, but at least she appeared to be listening to me. I turned over on my side and held my breath.

"No don't do that, just try and relax." She was quick in her application. I must say the results came fast and furious. I got into the bathroom as fast as I could move. This was not fun. I haven't had any surgery since I was a little girl. I think I was about six or seven years old. I had to have my tonsils removed and even then I wasn't alone. My cousins, Steve and Walter, both went in to have their tonsils removed at the same time. This was an all new experience for me. Facing the unknown alone.

Did I mention already that I was scared about out of my mind? I walked out of the bathroom and the little Spanish girl was just leaving the room. Before I could get my entire body back on the bed, in came another one of those traveling beds with two nurses pushing it. "It's time to go," the younger nurse said.

"Right now?"

"Yes," was the quick reply.

"Will someone tell my daughter where I am when she comes to visit me early this morning? She will be worried to death if I am not here in the room."

"Yes, I will see that someone informs her of the surgery," the younger nurse replied.

"I'm confused. The doctor told me in would be later in the morning. Somewhere around eleven o'clock."

"Well, that is possible, but he did change it, and you are to be downstairs in surgery by 6:30."

"Can't say I didn't try? I said with a slight smile.

Once in the elevator, the button was pushed for the bottom floor. My favorite. *"Oh please God, don't let me die in the basement," I prayed.* This time I was taken to another area where there were numerous other patients waiting in the hall on their traveling beds. Confusion seemed to be the order of the day. *This does not look promising. Several young doctors dressed in their scrubs were laughing and joking. Not at all what you would picture for a hospital setting. Some of the doctors were sitting on benches, changing their shoes. I remember one young girl, taking off a pair of clogs and replacing them with sneakers." Plus loud music was playing. Not elevator music, but hard rock. This is not promising at all.*

I was ushered into a small side room and left there, totally alone. Where the hell am I? And where the hell is this place?" I thought. I attempted to sit up and was suddenly but gently pushed back down on the Gurney.

"Hello," I am your anesthesiologist. My name is Doctor Hanson, and I will be putting you to sleep during the surgery.

"Would you please make sure that I go to sleep "Before" the surgery doc? "I would like that much better."

He smiled and said, "I can do that. I just wanted to introduce myself to you and let you know that I will be standing right along side of you during the procedure. Are you ready?"

"Do I have a choice?" I asked.

"Nope, lets go."

The operating room was small but it looked just like what you see in the movies and on tv. Bright lights and busy people. They slid me onto the table and began to strap me down in the stirrups. I could feel the heat of the lights above me and my heart was racing. I looked down at the floor to get my eyes off the lights when I noticed the doctors feet again. They all had sneakers on under their little blue or green scrub shoes. I turned to ask Dr. Hanson the question, when was he going to put me to sleep, but the words never made it out. Whatever was being pumped in my arm sure worked fast.

The first thing I remember doing upon awakening was to look at the clock on the wall. For a moment I had no idea where I was, or even what day it was. I heard a voice to the side of me say, "Oh young lady, your awake. How are you feeling?'

"Fine." The word came out before I could even think about my response. Funny thing was, I meant it. I really felt fine.

"Well that's just wonderful. I am going to be taking you back to your room, but first can I get you a drink of water?

"Please, that would be very nice, my throat feels very dry."

She returned with a small paper cup filled with cold water. "Here you go my dear. We be back in your room in just a few short minutes. The nurses stationed called and said your daughter was looking for you."

"I hope that they told her where I was. She would be frantic if she couldn't find me."

"Yes, they did and she is waiting for you in your room. So just relax and enjoy the ride on the elevator."

I saw Rah right away. There she was, just as the elevator door opened. I could see her looking in my direction. I started to wave both my arms, and yelled "Hello." "She smiled at me and then began to wave and run toward me.

"Well Rah, I made it this far, I said as I took a hold of her hand."

"Oh Mom, I have been here for over an hour and I was getting so nervous. But you look wonderful. How are you feeling?

"I really feel good. Whatever they put in me, really works. I haven't felt this good in over a year. She smiled her beautiful smile again, and we went through the doorway into my room.

The first thing I did when I got into my bed, was to push the Nurses call button. "Could I please have something to eat?"

There was a short pause and then a voice answered, "I'll check Mrs. Ayer. I will let you know."

43

"I will go out and get you something from the deli around the corner from the hospital, if you want me to Mom? It will only take me a few minutes."

"No, that's just silly. Let's see what they say before you do anything like that."

A few moments passed when there was a tap at the door. It was a nurse, she had a tray of food in her hands. She placed on the traveling tray and swung it in front of me. "I hope you like it."

"If you need anything else, just buzz."

"Oh thank you!" I removed the cover and saw the most beautiful turkey sandwich I had even seen. It seemed as if days had passed since I had eaten anything that even resembled solid food. I can't describe how wonderful that sandwich tasted. But I will never forget it, even if I live to be 90 years old. It tasted that good. Thank the Lord for small favors.

Rah sat very quietly in the corner and waited until I had finished eating before she started to ask questions. Most of her questions were in regard to the biopsy. What did I remember and how was it?

"I went right to sleep, and don't remember anything, Ra."

"Well that is a good thing," Rah replied smiling.

"I was just scared and nervous Rah. I remember that."

We were just relaxing and talking when my doctor walked into the room. "Mrs. Ayer, I am releasing you this afternoon, if you think that you are up to going home?" Dr. Johnson replied.

"Up to it? I am on my way home right now."

He smiled and said, "Now about the biopsy.

Oh here it comes, I thought.

" I already know. You don't have to say it. What is the prognoses?"

"I don't feel that a hysterectomy is necessary," he replied. I want you to call the "Woman's Cancer Center of RI first thing tomorrow morning and set up an appointment. My office and colleagues are there. We will discuss everything as soon as you feel that you are up to coming in. Here is the telephone number. Make sure you make the call tomorrow. "Treatment should begin immediately."

"I promise doctor, I will call." He turned and left the room without saying another word.

"Oh Mom, I prayed so hard that this was all a big mistake. It can't be true." Rah was crying very hard now.

"Lets not lose it at this point Rah. Lets find out exactly what can be done and how we are going to approach it. I need you Ra, so please stay with me here. Let's get packed and move our butts out of here before someone changes their mind.

"I'll call Nana, and let her know that they have released you and we are coming to her house right now," Rah said trying to dry her eyes.

Chapter 12
Home? What Home?

As Rah and I walked out of the automatic doors downstairs, I refused to look back. I had to make my self look toward the future. My life was on a new road. Perhaps a side street, perhaps a dead end. But I was going to give it my best. I had no idea what was ahead for me, but I had faith that it was the path that God wanted me to walk. And if the direction was not to my liking, that was just too bad. Not my will but thy will. So forward Pam, and think about it tomorrow.

On the way to my parents house, we stopped and both bought an ice coffee. Boy, did I miss my coffee. I am truly a coffee addict. Yes, I know that it is bad for me, but it's the little things right now that will get me through the day.

Mom and Dad both came to the door before I had time to ring the door bell. They must have been watching out the window for us. They both looked very tired and stressed. I wish I could spare them all this pain, and if it is within my power, that is exactly what I planned to do. I don't know how yet, but I will come up with something.

Before I could get my coat off, my mother started asking questions. "What are you going to do Pam, you can't go home? Not in your condition and with everything going on. You have to stay right here until this whole mess gets straightened out."

"How can I do that Mom?" I have only a few weeks to get all my belongings out of the house before it gets turned over to the bank. You know that the bank is going to foreclose, and I can't get any more extensions no matter what the excuse. I am going to have to put an ad in the paper and hopefully everything big will get sold and I will have a little money to show for my life.

As things stand right now, I don't even know where I am going to live. I have no money coming in, and now I have to worry about my health.

"Well, its plain that you are just going to have to live with your father and me and besides, there still could be some kind of mistake, you know. The doctors aren't really sure. They do make mistakes."

"Oh Mom, yes they are sure and so am I. You are going to have to face it. It's better to know than to be guessing all the time. Maybe now something will be done to improve my health. We have to look at it in that way. Think positive! I am going to call first thing tomorrow morning, and set up an appointment at the Cancer Center for Women. We will know a lot more after my appointment tomorrow. I am positive that my doctor will be able to give me some sort of idea of what kind of treatment I will be receiving." My mom turned silent and so did Rah. The silence lasted for what seemed like forever. You could truly hear a pin drop.

Rah finally broke the silence with, "I have to get going home now. The kids will be home and I have got to cook supper. Do you need anything at all Mom?"

"No, I am fine right now. You go and attend to your family. Please tell the kids hello for me." She gave me a quick hug, along with I'll call you later, and then she was gone.

Chapter 13
Parents and Kids

My mom and dad lived in a Senior Citizens Housing development which was operated by HUD. The apartments were very nice and clean and so were the grounds. But, what was most important, the rent was cheap. Both my parents had worked all their lives but only had Social Security to live on. Neither one had worked for a company offering retirement benefits. What a terrible shame. They both had worked so hard and here they were, forced to live in a one bedroom apartment about the size of their kitchen in their old home. The rules and regulations prohibited anyone staying at their residence for any length of time over two weeks. The office for the complex was directly across the street from them and the close surrounding of the other buildings prevented you from trying to get away with anything. Trying to stay with my parents could cause them some serious problems and could jeopardized their ability to remain there.

Considering what my options were, left me staying with one of my children. This was a very scary option for me. It wasn't that I didn't love them all, because I did. But I know that it would cause tension in their lives with their mates. Two women can not be in the kitchen at the same time. Not without some major problems. Plus who wants to live with their mother-in-law? Not very many. Especially a mother-in-law that is sick . What young couple trying to raise a family needs a cancer patient to complicate their lives anymore than they already all. And if I am going to be totally honest here, I don't want to cause any tension know just how stable any of my children's marriages are right now.

I know that Rah would love to have me with her. And I know that Brandon and Jason would as well. Afer all, I am their mother, but their mates? That is the question of the day. It was hard for me to think of all this. I would have given anything at this moment to find a closet big enough for me to crawl into and cry. But that was not even available to me. No closet would have held me in this little apartment. The thought of me trying to squeeze into one of them did bring a smile to my face. I would certainly have looked pretty stupid stuck in the doorway of one of them.

I had many phones calls that day. Mostly family, but my friend Joan called. She was my best friend and we had worked together for many years. She was divorced and had two grown children. Good kids, and very good to their mom. She had met Robert shortly after her divorce and they had been living together ever since. I think it is over six years now. Why they never have gotten married is anyone's guess, but they were happy with the way things were going. So just leave well enough alone.

"No Joan, there is nothing that you can do. It's just a waiting game right now, but I will call you and let you know what road I will be traveling."

"She replied, Oh sure you will!"

"If anyone knew me, it was Joan. No, I really promise. Thanks for calling and tell everyone at the post office I said hello." I hung up the phone and thought, *well at least there is one friend that really cares. The post office is a funny place. Everyone is so busy trying to move up that real friendships are rare. People have short memories sometimes. Once they reach their desired position, they forget your name. I have to stop thinking about the past. I must try and take each moment as they come.*

My dad cooked his speciality. His wonderful spaghetti. He knows how much I love it. I must say it tasked even more delicious than I remembered. My mom and dad went to bed early, as they always do and I was left with the couch. I didn't mind. I was mentally tired, not physically tired. So I just laid back and relaxed with the tv remote in my hand and began to surf the channels for a horror movie. It didn't matter to me if it was a good one or a bad one. I had most likely already seen it. The objective was to keep my mind off tomorrow and the bank repossession. I propped a pillow under my legs and took some deep cleansing breaths. The pillows seemed to help me before, so I thought "I'll give them a try tonight." I had just located the Wolfman on the Sci-Fi channel, when my eyes began to get heavy. I must have seen this one at least a hundred times. That was my last thought before I fell asleep.

49

Chapter 14
Treatment

Bright sunlight came into the living room, and my eyes opened slowly. Now where am I?, was the first thought that appeared in my brain. But it only took a second or two when I recognized the surroundings. I slept surprising well on the old couch. The pills I had taken the night before, had a lot to do with my uninterrupted rest. "I wonder if I will ever sleep in my own bed again?" I will probably find out the answer to that question very soon. I just wish I knew how long I had (Oh that doesn't sound good) before I had to sell everything? But, first things first. Cancer is the first mountain to climb, the furniture will have to be second and if I have to, I will give it away to my kids. I began to feel sorry for myself. Which I have been doing often lately, and I hate myself for doing it. What did I do to deserve this? I don't just mean the cancer, I mean everything. Did I do something terrible in my life, and I am being punished? I can't say that I remember ever deliberately hurting anyone in my life. Either I had selective memory, or I just truthfully had never hurt anyone on purpose. But, only God knows for sure.

Dad was the first one up and moving around. He usually was, that was just his way. "Morning Pam, how are you doing, and did you get any sleep?"

"Yes, I slept pretty good Dad. Are you going to cook, I am really feeling hungry?" "Whatever you want, just tell me. Do you want some eggs and bacon?"

"Oh goodness no, just some toast Dad. I don't know what they are going to do to me today, so I am going to eat light this morning."

"Well you stay right where you are, and I will fix it for you."

That's my dad for you. Always so thoughtful. I don't think that he is capable of a selfish thought. It was just not his way. Truly a fine man and a gentleman. I relaxed and got comfortable. Just let me get over this hurdle, I will do one hurdle at a time. After all, I am not still in the hospital. My treatments will most likely be as an outpatient. Oh, treatments. Most likely Chemo. I don't know much about it, but I know that it's not pleasant. At least that is what I have heard. Get your mind off it now Pam. You still have a lot to be thankful for. I looked around the room, the room was small and filled with the small amount of old furniture my parents had, but they were content. Now me, here I was 54 years old, divorced and having my elderly father and mother take care of me. Was I never going to grow up? And yet I felt lucky and thankful that I still had both of my parents with me. So many of my friends had lost either their mom or their dad or even both. My parents were still here and in good health.

I took a few moments to give thanks for these gifts and all the other gifts that were given to me. The important ones were still with me. It is important for me to take the time to be thankful for those things. Yes, I am losing material things, and my health is on the shaky side right now but I am not without the love of my family. That should be more important than anything else.

My mom got up shortly and we talked. I told her that first on my list was to call the Women Cancer Center for my appointment. I had to find out what was my future so that I could start dealing with the bank and the post office, plus finding a place to live while all this stuff was happening. This was truly a challenge. I had always been good with challenges. I never liked to give up on anything. I had come to grips that moving was inevitable. But one thing was not in that picture was that I was not going to be able to work and earn some money. I already had planned on selling most of my furniture (I had a seventeen room house filled with it, including a pool table) and using that cash along with my paycheck to have enough money for the first, last, and security deposit on an apartment somewhere. Wrong! The way things were looking, I was not even going to be able to keep my car. My Eagle Talon. And yes, I was in the category of one of those people who loved their cars. What's that saying? "So sad, too bad?" Just how did things get so out of hand?

Rah called early and was just checking that I was going to make the call to the doctors.

"Yes daughter dear, I am going to call as soon as I hang up with you. I will call you back and let you know what the plan is." My hands were shaking when

I picked up the telephone. My voice cracked when the voice on the other end said, "Woman's Cancer Center." How can I help you?"

Help me? I thought. How about telling me it was all a mistake and I don't really have cancer. Instead I politely said, I need to make an appointment with Dr. Johnson as soon as possible.

"Would tomorrow morning at eight be alright for you?"

" That would be fine. I'll be there." She gave me the directions on exactly where the building was located and instructed me to go to the second floor (I don't care for the number 2 at all) I wrote all the directions down and relayed the information to my mom and dad. Of course you know that they were staring at me and listening to the entire conversation.

Well, at least I can rest today. I am not even going to get dressed. My pain was at the pounding level and I knew that it was time for another pain killer. "I am going with you tomorrow," my Mom said firmly.

"I assumed you would want to go. I do want you to go with me Mom, so don't get excited. Just promise me that you will let me do the talking. Okay?"

"Well, I think we should write all the questions down before we get there. Ada says you won't forget anything important if you write it down first. (Ada was a close friend of my mothers who lived in the apartment right above my parents) She was an old maid and had lived there for over 40 years. She had moved in with her elderly mother to take care of her, and when her mother passed away she kept the apartment. I am not positive, but I think Ada is close to being 95 years old. She still has all her facilities but is a classic busy body.

"Mom, why don't you write down all the things you want to know for now, and I will think of some of the questions I want answered. Later on when I feel a little better, we can go over them? I think that it is a very good idea," I said. That made her smile.

I slept the rest of the morning. I think I was a tad high. So many medications and my body was not used to any of them. Zombie land is where I visited every time I took them. So you can understand why I keep losing track of time. Rah came in but I don't know when. She was in the kitchen with my parents when I awoke from my little nap.

"Hi sleepy head," She said.

I smiled at her and said, "Do I know you?" She burst out laughing. Rah always had a great sense of humor, and I could usually manage to get a giggle out of her.

"What are you guys talking about?" my mom asked.

"Well," Rah replied. "The Questions," and started to giggle.

"Oh the "Questions." This my mom did not think was funny at all. Of course Rah and I both were really laughing at this point.

"Now just stop it you two, this is serious."

"I know Ma, I'm sorry. Just let me tease you a little. It makes me feel better. You know I love you." That was the wrong thing to say. My mother started crying immediately. "Now stop mom." Let me see what you have for questions."

To my surprise they had created a great list. What type of treatment will I be having? What are the side effects? What is the duration of the treatment and especially what is the prognosis? "Well, those are all the main questions, I think you covered all the major points. Thank you. I know that I will be so nervous, I might not even be able to open my mouth."

The phone rang, and I motioned to my mom that I did not want to talk to anyone, at least not right now. "No, she is sleeping right now, can I have her call you back? Yes, thanks for calling and I will tell her you called when she wakes up. Pam, that was Joe from the Silvertown post office. He just wanted you to know that everyone is praying for you." I knew the news wouldn't take long to spread. What's it been, a day and a half? Bad thoughts again. I must stop it. They are just being nice. The Silvertown office has some very nice people working there. I am just judging them because of a few bad apples.

The rest of the day I continued to doze on and off. Brandon and Susan, stopped by later in the evening and they had the girls with him. Alex was nine years old and was lovely and very outspoken. "Meme, please don't die." Apparently her little friends grandmother had just died from cancer. This must of frightened her terribly.

"Don't worry pumpkin, Meme is going to do everything she can do to get better. I am not going to leave you. God will take care of me, so you just say a little prayer for me every night and that will help me to get well."

Brianna (who is seven years old) spoke up. "I will pray too, and my daddy is going to make you a place to live in my house. We will take care of you, so don't worry Meme."

"Well, that would be nice Bri. I appreciate the offer."

Susan quickly stopped Bri from saying anything else. "Please don't be upset Pam, Susan replied. We love you, and we want you with us. We can take care of you. We want to help. Our house is plenty big enough and you should not be left alone."

"Thank you again. It is very comforting to know that you want to help. I will know a lot more tomorrow." Brandon gathered up his family and I promised to call them sometime later. This decision was definitely the one I suspected was being discussed in the cafeteria during my stay in the hospital when they all went downstairs together… I may be sick, but I am not stupid.

Once they left, I settled back onto the couch. I had a lot to think about again. Just the decisions were draining my strength.

Chapter 15
Women's Cancer Center

I had a restless night and was extremely tired when the sun came up. Strangely enough, I was feeling calm. Perhaps I knew the answers where close. I can't solve a problem with out knowing exactly where I stand. In a strange way, the cancer diagnosis was a relief. At least I knew what was wrong with me. Maybe it can be fixed, maybe not. But before long the questions would be answered.

I showered, once again using the steel bars on the wall for support, and let the tears begin. This was my safe place. No one could see me cry. I didn't have to pretend in here. Slowly the tears ceased. I stepped out of the shower and I approached the mirror, I was pitiful looking. You could see every bone in my body. I looked like I had anorexia. My face was so sunken and sallow colored. I don't think I weighed 100 pounds at this point.

What the heck was I going to wear. Most of my clothes were at my house. Nothing fits me anymore especially the ones Rah had packed in the suitcase. I know, I thought. *I will wear my dads red sweatshirt that my mother had shrunk. I will put my white blouse under it and wear my black sweat pants. Sweat pants always look baggy on everybody. I finished my hair and did my best with my makeup. The results were not great, but they will have to do. Besides, who knows me where I am going?*

I had a light breakfast, (toast, juice and coffee) with my mom. I wasn't sure if I should eat anything, but I had to keep something in me or I would get sick again. I didn't want that to happen. Rah arrived and we climbed into her car and headed for the unknown territory of Cancer Land.

The drive to Providence was took about ten minutes. The building was very easy to find. The secretary had given great directions. The building was brick, not excessively large, with many windows. My guess would be about three or four stories high. They had a parking lot directly across from the hospital where I had been just a couple of days before. Rah parked the car and we all got out with tension written all over our faces. Rah took my hand, and I took my moms hand and into the front doors we walked.

The lobby was lovely. Lots and lots of flowering plants and a beautiful fountain right in the center of the room. We stepped into the elevator, which was the size of a cracker jacks box, and I pushed button # 2 (Ugh, bad number) The door opened and we all walked out as a family.

A receptionist was seated right in front of the elevator doors. She was a tiny little thing with blonde hair. She looked up and smiled beautifully at us. I gave my name and she scanned her appointment book. She stood up from her desk and said, "if you will follow me Ms. Ayer." She led us into one of the prettiest waiting areas I have ever seen. All the furnishings were French Provincial. There was a very large screen tv, lovely drapes, fresh flowers and all sorts of Women magazines on the coffee tables. There were six couches with brocade fabric and matching throw pillows on the side. "If you would like to take a seat, the doctor should be arriving shortly." I glanced at Rah and I knew that she was thinking the same as me. Boy, this is fancy!

I must have had one of the first appointments of the day as their were no other patients in the waiting area. So, we had our choice of which lovely couch we wanted to sit on. I picked up a magazine trying to look like I was somewhat relaxed. But my heart was racing. What was beyond those doors? Through those two doors was the answer to my life. Will I live or will I die? Just how strong and how much courage did I have inside me. I knew that the answer was not far way.

We sat for a short time and one by one the ladies, the young girls and the children all came in. Some had no hair, some had hats on, and others were wearing wigs. A young girl about the age of thirteen sat directly across from me and next to her was her mother. "Your new here aren't you? she asked.

I smiled and said, "Yes I am. Does it show?"

"It's your hair, I can tell you haven't had any treatments yet." she replied. You'll do just fine. Besides, it's not always bad. You will have some good days, and sometimes you will be sick. But try not to worry, I have been coming for my chemo for four months now. What kind of cancer do you have?" At that

56

question, her mother gave her a gentle poke and a very disapproving look. "I am sorry, I shouldn't have asked that."

Her mother interrupted her and said "Please forgive my daughter, she is very forward sometimes."

"It's quite alright. I have cervical cancer. I was just diagnosed a few days ago."

"I have leukemia. The doctor says I have a long way to go, but I seem to be getting better." Her mother smiled and said, "Yes she has improved greatly. We are very positive regarding her recovery."

I smiled and returned to my magazine. Another lump in my throat had materialized and I was fighting back the tears.

An older woman, in her late 50's, approached me and held out her hand. "You must be Mrs Ayer?"

"Yes, I am," I replied.

"Please come with me, as I would like to show you around the facility. Your family may come too, if they like." All three of us stood up and I introduced Rah and my mother.

"I am sorry, I forgot to introduce myself. I am Liz Walker. It's very nice to meet you all. Now if you will follow me. I will give you the grand tour."

We approached the "Doors." I held my breath as we passed through them. I could see desks and a few offices enclosed with glass. "This is the Secretarial unit. All the paperwork such as medical reports, billing, and etc. for each patient, is done right here. In back of the desks, through the door that has the window, are the individual medical records. She turned to the right and we walked through a narrow hallway. There were four more rooms off this hallway. She stopped at each room, and brought me inside them, showing me what the room contained. They were all about the same size. Two of the rooms had full size beds, tv's and bathrooms. The other two were designed like a living room. Each had a recliner, with two other comfortable chairs and a tv, VCR, a radio, and telephones. Plus full bathrooms. "You can see that everything is designed to allow you to be as comfortable as possible. You can also receive a body massage and any thing you would like to eat during your treatments. We left these rooms and walked a short distance down the hall. In the next room was a full kitchen. Including a refrigerator, stove sink and cupboards full of food. I believe the food was prepared for you while you were in treatment. My amazement was evident by the expression on my face. Ms. Walker just smiled and continued on with the tour. We turned and retraced our steps to the secretarial section. We walked to our left and saw the six exam rooms.

Located In the center of these exam rooms stood the Doctors station. My guess would be this is where they consulted with each other regarding their patients. Mrs Walker also pointed out the Doctors lounge and their cafeteria. "We have our own laboratory downstairs where all your blood work will be done."

"Do you have any questions?"

"No, it's very nice and not at all what I had expected."

"We pride ourselves in making every woman who comes here as comfortable as humanly possible. If you will follow me one more time, I will bring you back to the reception area. I will be seeing you again, Ms Ayer and good luck." She shook my hand, smiled and walked away. I sat down on the couch and noticed that the young girl was gone. I only had to wait a few more minutes before my name was called. We all rose from the couch and followed the woman who had the clip board in her hand. She brought us to exam room # 6 (another even number, ugh) and instructed me to get undressed and get on the table. The doctor would be in momentarily. I did as I was instructed and picked up the dressing gown and headed for the bathroom. Once inside I sat down on the toilet and thought, *Hold it together, Pam. God, how I hate those stirrups.* I removed my clothes, and put the dressing gown on and walked back into the exam room. My mom and Rah had seated themselves in the corner of the room. Before I could say anything to them, Dr. Johnson came into the room.

"Good morning, Ms. Ayer."

"Good morning, Doctor."

"Let me get right to the point. You are going to lose all your hair."

"My hair, I don't care about my hair, I said with a touch of sarcasm. Doctor, what about the tumor?"

"After reviewing the results of the biopsy and all the other tests, I have come to the conclusion that you have a stage four tumor in your vagina. There was some consideration of removing your uterus and ovaries, but at this point, I don't believe that is necessary. The tumor is very well advanced, but has confined itself to the wall of your vagina. At this point there is no sign of any spread of cancer in other regions in your body. I want to start you on Chemotherapy and radiation as fast as possible. My nurse will give you the address of two different radiation centers in RI. Both are excellent. It will be your choice on which one you would prefer. Naturally your Chemo will take place here. My secretary will also set up your first chemo session. It is of most importance that you make the phone call regarding the radiation. As both treatments compliment the other. We have had excellence results with this kind of tumor using the combination of both Chemo and radiation. Do you have any questions?"

Rah spoke right up. "How long will the treatments be?"

"If you mean how long they take, about five or six hours each visit. If you mean the entire course of treatment, with success there is the possibility of eight or nine months. And that is just an estimate." I almost fell off the exam table. Eight or nine months? I couldn't believe it. Why did I think that this was going to be a quick process. Why, because I was stupid. I hadn't given it any thought. None! I don't know why I could have let this escape my thoughts.

"I don't feel as if an exam is necessary today, Ms. Ayers. You can get dressed now. Make sure you stop by the front desk for those address and make your first appointment." He turned and left the room. I was still in total shock. *My thoughts went to yesterday, when I should have been reading everything I could get my hands on regarding cervical cancer instead of just lying around all day.*

I got off the exam table and walked toward the bathroom to change my clothes. "I looked at Rah, and said, "I don't want to talk right now, but I am alright." I closed the door of the bathroom and turned the water on and flushed the toilet, all the while holding on to the sink just crying. I gathered myself together and got dressed and returned to Rah and Mom who were standing at the door.

We walked to the secretaries desk, and she promptly gave me the list that Dr. Johnson had mentioned and then set up my first appointment for one week from today. I couldn't help myself and said, "Oh boy, I can hardly wait." I folded the piece of paper she had given to me and placed it in my pocket. "Okay, lets go." When we reached the car, I still had not said anything. My mind was a little preoccupied. Once all seat belted in, I turned to Rah and said, "That was a barrel of laughs, lets do it again one week from today." I started to laugh. Rah joined in quickly. There we were in the parking lot of a cancer center laughing our heads off. My mother did not see the humor in any of it. "Mom, you have to learn to laugh, it's the only way to true love and peace of mind." She looked at me as if I had lost my mind. Poor Mom, she just didn't understand me, not even now. If I couldn't laugh, I wouldn't be able to survive.

We stopped and got some coffee on the way home. Conversation was at a minimum to say the least.

Chapter 16
Decisions

By the time we got back to the my parents apartment it was almost noontime. Dad was standing in the kitchen when we walked in. "How did it go?" "What did you find out?'

"Oh dad, I have to have chemotherapy and radiation. And it looks like it is going to take a long time to get better."

"Oh," was his reaction. But his hand were holding on to the stove tightly.

"But the good news is it looks like the cancer stayed in one place. That is a big plus for me. We have that to be thankful for." I went to put my hand in my pocket and felt the piece of paper the secretary had given me. *I should call one of these numbers right away,* I thought. I walked over and sat down in my moms' rocker and read the piece of paper. The first treatment center listed was in the Providence Hospital. The second one was in Fairfield right across the street from the County Hospital. I knew exactly where it was. This one was going to be my choice. Not only was it not inside a hospital, but it was only about one mile from my son Brandon's house.

I told Rah about what I had read and told her that I was going to choose the one in Fairfield. I knew the treatment one in the hospital was closer but I would have to pay for parking and I did not want to enter the hospital again for any reason. Fairfield was farther away, but was in a better environment for me. I am going to call and make the appointment right now. I reached for the phone and dialed the number. Fairfield Oncology and Radiation, This is Jean."

"Hi Jean, my name is Pamela Ayer, and I have been referred to you by Dr.

CRYING IN THE SHOWER - CERVICAL CANCER

Johnson for treatments."

"Oh yes, we are very familiar with Dr. Johnson. We see many of his patients. Would you like to come in tomorrow for a consultation, say about one in the afternoon?"

"Yes, that would be fine," I answered.

"Could you spell your last name again?"

"A Y E R, " I replied.

"Do you know the findings of Dr Johnson, Ms. Ayer?"

"Yes, Cervical Cancer. I have a tumor in my vagina."

"Alright I will call Dr. Johnson's office right now, and have him Fax a record of his tests over here right away. We will see you tomorrow. "Bye and thank you for calling."

I put the phone down and took another one of my deep breaths. Now that's taken care of, I thought. Tomorrow at one. Onward and Upward Pam. There is no stopping me now. What could be next?

Mom was sitting next to Rah on the couch. "I just don't think I can handle this. It should be me, not my daughter. I want to die right now. I can't take it."

"Mom, please don't start this. We all take our turns and this time it is mine."

"Well its not fair, Rah added. You have enough problems. You don't deserve this."

"Who does deserve it Rah? The little girl who sat across from us or maybe someone else in the waiting area with us?"

"Mom, I didn't mean it that way. You know that."

"I know you didn't, but we have to think clear and concentrate on the things that we can control. We can't control what is happening with the cancer. That is in Gods control and with help from the doctors, things will work out. Let's move on to another subject for now. How about some food? I'm feeling better and I know I should eat something. What's is the kitchen that's hot and delicious?"

My father smiled and said, "Whatever you desire, I will cook it."

What a man. Why couldn't I find myself one like him? That was the question that haunted me. Why on earth did I pick the one I did? I don't want to think about him. Change the subject in your mind, Pam.

I called Brandon next. "Thank you for calling Fast Lube, this is Brandon, how can I help you?" "I laughed, "This is your mother, and I have returned from my adventure at the doctors. Do you have a minute that you can talk or is it too busy there?"

"Of course I can talk, I'm the boss. How did you make out, mom?"

61

"Not great, I have to have chemo and radiation treatments starting right away. Silence on the other end. Brandon, are you still with me?"

"Yeah, will they be able to get all the cancer?"

"That part I think is good. It didn't spread and hopefully the treatments will be successful. But here is the main reason that I called. My radiation treatments are going to be right near your house. I have to go there tomorrow afternoon. I was thinking that I will go over to your house when I get done. We can talk more about it then. Is that okay?

"Where near my house, Mom?"

"It's right across the street from the County Hospital. So you don't have to bother coming over here tonight. Call me later on this evening, if you want. Bye for now, I love you"

"Love you too, ma. Bye."

Chapter 17
Radiation Time

My night was filled with dreams. Not pleasant ones. Machines and sounds and green scrubs all around me. When I awoke, I felt more tired than before I had gone to sleep. I had tossed and turned (not easy of the couch) constantly. I could not find anything interesting on the tv. Wouldn't you think with over 200 channels a person could find something worth while to watch? I finally managed to fall asleep somewhere between a muscle bound man selling an exercise machine and another man dressed in a suit selling a sure fire get rich scheme using a computer.

I sat up and regretted it almost immediately. I don't know how the muscles and nerves are connected in your body, but the tumor was pushing on my back, my rear end and my lower extremities. I was a mess. My high tolerance of pain was beginning to weaken.

My mom was in the kitchen. "You actually beat dad and your up first?" I asked.

"Oh no, he has been up for at least an hour." He is taking his usual walk around the complex and then he was going to the market to buy some pancake mix. He insisted that he was going to make you pancakes this morning."

"God love him. I'll never be as healthy as him when I reach his age, if I reach his age."

The phone rang. "Hello," I said.

"Hi Mom, its Jay. How are you doing?"

"Okay, I am glad you called."

"What is going on today?" he asked.

"I am going to the Radiation Doctor this afternoon."

"Is there anything Ann and I can do for you?"

"Not right now, son. I'll call you later on this afternoon and let you know how I make out."

"Mom, I love you."

"I know that Jay, don't worry. I am going to get through this. You tell Ann and Cheyenne that I said hello."

" I will, and don't forget to call me later as soon as you find out anything," Jay asked politely.

"I promise. Bye for now, son."

"Bye mom."

"Pam, do you need a pill? My mom asked.

"No I better not. I want to eat something first. Is there any coffee?"

"Of course, your father made it first thing this morning. Do you want me to make a fresh pot?" my mom asked.

"If you wouldn't mind," I replied.

"I'll try, but you know that this is your fathers job."

"I know, " and smiled at her. Dad did do everything around the house. Mom was not exaggerating with that statement.

I had to go to the bathroom, but it seemed so far away and I hurt so bad. The worse part was besides the pain, I had diarrhea all the time. Good grief, I was a mess.

My Mom and I sat at the table and just talked for a little while. There were so many things I wished that I could say to my mother. I loved her so. She had always tried to be there for me. I didn't tell her I loved her very often at all. I believe that I held my words inside me just as she had taught me to. I was like her no matter how hard I fought it.

Gram was the one that would hug me and say the words I needed to hear as a child. She showed me how to love and how to accept my moms way. She would tell me every day, your mother loves you Pam. It's just her way, and she is ill right now.

For most of my childhood, my mom had many different health problems. My biological father had given her a disease when she was carrying a child. The results were disastrous and she lost the baby. The results from the infection were, she had to have myself and my brother by caesarian. She had some serious complications which resulted in a complete hysterectomy at the young age of 32. There were no hormones in those days, and the shock to her body

CRYING IN THE SHOWER - CERVICAL CANCER

was extremely difficult for her to handle mentally. Plus there was a serious problem with the hysterectomy. She was sent home with a very serious infection which almost caused her death.

That is one of my earliest memories of my mom. She was in her bedroom, which was totally dark, with a man in a dark suit (a priest) giving her the last rites. I had no idea what was going on, I only wanted to talk to her and showed her that I could almost blow a bubble. with chewing gum. Silly isn't it? The things you remember. But how I cried when they wouldn't let me in to see her and show her my "almost bubble." Gram comforted me as usual. She was always there in those days. She was taking care of me and my brother plus my mom. I remember what she would tell me. "Pam, your not extraordinally beautiful, but you have a special beauty about you. Remember this, you are no better than anyone else in this world, but no one is better than you."

"If you can remember that and live by it, you will have a better life."

I lost Gram when she was 92 years old. I still miss her every day of my life. But I always feel that she is with me, guiding me along and giving me the strength that I need. I know that if this cancer takes me that she will be the first face I see in heaven.

My thoughts of Gram were interrupted with my dads whistling. He whistled constantly. But I don't think he even knew he was doing it. But it was a comforting sound.

"I got the pancake mix for you Pam. I hope your hungry?"

"You bet Dad. Cook away," I said smiling at him.

We sat down and enjoyed a nice breakfast together. Rah called and said she would be here around 12:30. Great, that will give me enough time to get ready. Still have to make a good impression and keep up a good front. Can't forget to smile.

Rah arrived right on schedule, only this time my Mom couldn't go with us. Haley was not feeling well and could not go to school. Mom was elected to stay with her because dad was not good taking care of sick kids. So it was just Rah and me headed for Fairfield and the radiation doctor.

We got there in plenty of time. Not much traffic and Rah knew exactly where it was. We both walked in to the front desk and I gave my name. Once again we sat in a waiting area. I thought that I would see a lot more patients, but there was only one other person sitting there. This time it was a man. We waited about fifteen minutes and a young nurse came and escorted myself and Rah into another exam room. (No number on this one) She instructed me to get undressed from the waist down and sit on the table. Dr. Merrick would be

65

right in. I looked at Rah and said, "You know I have had more men looking at me in my private parts in the past few days, than in my entire life. I am beginning to feel like I should start charging them and make some fast money. What do you think Rah?"

Her shocked look tickled the heck out of me. "Mom! Don't say such things." She then started to laugh right along with me.

Dr. Merrick opened the door. "Well, what's going on in here? he said smiling. I haven't heard laughter in one of my exam rooms in a long time. It's good to know that you have a solid sense of humor. It helps speed up the recovery process.

He looked like your typical hometown family physician. Overweight, grey hair, about 5'8" tall and a flushed complection. He smiled again, and I knew that I liked him right away. "I read your medical reports and the results of the biopsy. I really need to examine you, to see the tumor itself. This is going to be uncomfortable, but I will try and be as gentle as possible." He went over to the sink and put on some funny glasses. They looked like magnifying glasses three inches thick. Next came the rubber gloves. Oh boy, I thought. He pulled the little stool out and moved a high powered light over his shoulder. "Breath normally, now."

There was no exaggeration on his part. Yes it was very uncomfortable. Extremely painful. But it was over quickly. He went to the sink and removed the gloves and glasses and washed his hands. He leaned on the sink and folded his arms. "You certainly do have a very unusual type of tumor there. If you would get dressed and meet me in my office we can discuss the way will approach the treatment." He then left the room without saying anything else.

I got off the table and started to get dressed. "I like him Rah, what about you?"

"Me too, Mom. He is very down to earth. Lets go and see what he has to say. Are you okay mom, I know that it hurt you?"

"Well I am going to have to find a ladies room. I know I am bleeding again. But I am alright for the moment."

We walked to his office, just across from the exam room. I could see him sitting behind his desk. "My that was fast. I was just looking at the biopsy report." He pointed to the chair in front of his desk and I sat down. What I want to do is start treatment right away, without any delay. I need you to come in tomorrow for your beginning treatments. My associate will be coming in this evening and we shall plan out exactly how we are going to attack this tumor."

"What can I expect from radiation treatments?" I asked.

"Reactions vary from patient to patient. There is medication that will help with the side effects" So try not to concern yourself at this point. I am confident that we can destroy this tumor with systematic blasts of radiation plus the chemotherapy. But it will not be done overnight. I will know more after a few treatments. I will have to see how your body reacts to the treatments overall. How do you feel about this Mrs. Ayer?"

"I am totally overwhelmed at this point. Am I going to die from this?"

"Mrs. Ayer, everyone dies, we just don't know when and from what. Just stay positive." He stood up and shook my hand.

"Thank you, I will make the appointment on my way out."

I scheduled an appointment for eight 8 o'clock in the morning the next day. "Well Rah, all I can say right now, is that exam was the closest thing to sex that I have had in five years." We laughed all the way to the car.

Chapter 18
Brandon's Offer

The ride to Brandon's house took about five minutes. He had a lovely home which sat back off the main road. The yard was extremely well maintained with only a few leaves on the grass remained. These remaining leaves must have been caused by the cool fall weather we had been experiencing, as I know that Brando or Susan would not allow their yard to look unkept.

The house was a two story colonial. Dressed in green shutters with a large green front door. Susan was standing at the front door waiting for us. As we pulled in the driveway, Susan came out the front door. She smiled and invited us in.

"Your home looks so nice Susan, you and Brandon have done a lot of work."

"Never mind the house. Come on in, it is cold out here."

Their home was a show piece. Susan was truly gifted in decorating on a budget. I know what Brandon made for a salary, and Susan only had a part time job because of having to be home with the girls.

We entered the front door, to the left of the foyer was another door that led to the basement. Ahead of us was the stairway that brought you to the main living quarters. The basement was an exact replica of the upstairs only it was framed but totally unfinished, and used only for storage. The builder had meant to make the house a duplex, but for financial reasons the basement remained unfinished. In a way it worked out well for Brandon, as he was able to purchase the house for a very reasonable price.

We walked up the stairs with Susan acting very nervous. She was chattering, which is not one of her normal traits. "Brandon is on his way home.

He wants to talk to you, Pam."

I looked at her and asked, "Is this something I want to hear? I really can't take any more bad news right now."

"It's nothing like that Pam. It's just something that we have all come up with for your benefit. But for right now, tell me how it went at the doctors?"

I didn't go into very much detail, but I did try and tell her all the important parts.

"God Pam, this is just awful. How can you be so calm?"

"I am too sick to care, if you want me to be honest. There is nothing we can do about it, it's just one of those little things that happens in life. You never know when it will be your turn. After meeting Dr. Merrick today, I do feel more positive than I did yesterday. Dr Johnson has a tendency to be all gloom and doom. On the other side of the coin, Dr Merrick was much more upbeat. For what it's worth, he makes me feel quite comfortable and confident in him."

We sat at the kitchen and had coffee and some pie (in between my bathroom trips, can't forget them) and general conversation. I heard the down stairs front door open and within seconds two little voices rang out. "Meme" Up the stairs they ran, running side by side. There they were, two of the prettiest little girls you will ever see. Both of them had long, long dark hair and dark eyes. Alex's eyes were almond shaped like her moms and Brianna's eyes were round and large like her fathers. And yet if you looked at the two of them, you would think that they were twins. They both were extraordinarily beautiful.

"Oh Meme, I am so glad to see you, Alex cried." Her armed were wrapped around me in a heartbeat.

Bri was trying to squeeze her way in at the same time. "Me to, Meme" said Bri.

"Well not as happy as I am to see you. I feel better already just seeing you two." Big smiles crossed their little beautiful faces.

"Your coming to live with us, Bri blurted out.

"I am?"

"Yep, daddy is already working on your bedroom downstairs."

"Bri, that is enough" quipped Susan. We are waiting for your daddy to come home to talk about that."

Rah's face was serious, "Mom, don't say anything yet. Please wait until Brandon gets here before you make any decisions."

"Alright, I will, don't get nervous. I listen to what he has to say before I say a word."

"So how are my girls?"

"Fine" they said in unison."

"So tell me how school is? Do you have any boyfriends?"

"Oh Meme! You always ask us that. No, we don't have any boyfriends," Bri said giggling. "Well then are you engaged?"

"NO!!" Alex's answered totally discussed. I am too young."

I laughed and said, "You know that I love to tease you. But no getting married until you reach the age of 25. Promise me, now."

"Okay we promise," said Bri.

Alex had managed to get on my lap. She laid her head down on my chest and she sighed deeply. "I love you so much Meme."

"I love you too little one." She was pressing her head so hard on my chest that I was having trouble breathing. "Don't worry, Cat." (Alex's nickname) I am going to be around for a long, long time. Who else will tease you if I don't?"

She looked up at me and smiled. There is my little girl. Always keep that beautiful smile. It will make everyone around you happy and that is a very good thing. You have that special gift, you make sure you use it." She squeezed me one more time and then got down off my lap.

Susan instructed them to go to their bedroom for now until their father got home. "He should be here any minute. Susan and Rah talked about their kids and all the homework that the schools give them. Susan mentioned having to bring Alex to the library at least two times a week. "Oh that reminds me, I want to go to the library and get some books on Cervical cancer. I really need to look up all the information that is out there."

Sue quickly replied, "I'll take you the next time I bring Alex, if your up to it."

Rah frowned and replied, "I don't know if you should really do that Mom. It might scare you. You know that the doctors both said that each case is different."

"I know your right Rah, but I have to find out at least where this cancer came from, if nothing else."

We heard a car pull into the driveway and then a door slam. "Here comes Brandon," Sue stood up. She was right. Up the stairs he came like gangbusters. His long legs taking two stairs at a time easily.

"Hello mother," in his usual wise ass tone.

"Hello sonny boy," my usual wise ass answer. He pulled up a chair and threw his coat onto the couch. He immediately lit up a cigarette. Oh I thought to myself, this is going to be fun.

"Mom, Susan and I and Rah have been talking. We feel that you would be much better here while you are so sick rather than at Nana's. Rah would take you to live with her, but with the four kids you would be far from comfortable and you would have no privacy. She does not have an extra bedroom for you. You would be on the couch again. That is not where someone going through cancer treatments should be. How would you get any rest? How does this sound? You stay at Rah's house over each weekend for your Chemo treatments and then come here and stay for your radiation treatments. I know that this depends on how many days a week you need the Chemo and radiation treatments. But what do you think?"

"Well, we don't have all the information yet regarding the treatments, but where am I going to sleep Brandon? You don't have any extra bedrooms either.

"Come with me, Mom." Brandon stood up and walked over to me. "Can you manage going downstairs?

"Oh yes, I took a pill when I had the coffee." He took my arm and guided me to the stairway with everyone following. Alex and Bri came running out of their bedroom, I am sure that they were listening at their door. The little devils.

We walked downstairs and he opened the door to the basement. On the floor was a pile of sheet rock with nails, hammers, and all sorts of other carpenter tools. We turned to the right and there was another door. A new door. Brandon opened the door and inside was a room totally carpeted, and sheet rocked. The ceiling tile was completely finished and, all the electrical outlets were installed. A new ceiling fan and a new set of double closet doors were installed for a new clothes closet and with precision placed properly into the wall. Shock does not properly describe what I felt.

"When did you do all this Brandon, and where did you get the money?"

" I have been working night and day on this Mom. I will be putting in a bath, a kitchen plus a living room. You will have a separate entrance all your own. We will be upstairs if you need us, and if you want privacy it will be here for you downstairs. As for the money part, I will do a little bit at a time. Whenever we have extra money. What do you think?"

I was at a total loss for words. Tears filled my eyes.

"Mom we all talked it over and this is really the best thing for you right now, Rah added. Of course it will depend on the treatments, but I think that this will work out nicely for you."

As we returned upstairs, no one said a word. I had a lot to think about. It is true that I had always gotten along fine with Susan. If I had the separate living quarters I wouldn't be intruding on her territory. I love and girls and enjoyed

71

their company very much, so I knew that wouldn't be a problem. Also, there was no question in my mind regarding my son. I loved him and we were as close as any mother and son could be. I felt that way about all my children. I loved them all with all my heart. True, they all had totally different personalities, and sometimes I wondered how three children with the same mother and father could be so different, but that was just the way they were. So, for now all I could do was wait and see what the cancer had planned for me. But this idea of Brandon's just might be the answer to where I was going to live.

"Just give me a little time to think it over. There's a lot to be considered. I have had a tough day, and I really need to get some rest."

Chapter 19
Realization Strikes

Rah drove me back to my parents apartment and it was decided on the way home, that none of what had occurred at Brandon's house would be mentioned to either of them. I am pretty sure that dad would say, "you do what you think is best" and let it go as that. But my mother was another story. She had never been fond of Susan or any of Susan's family. But I believe that her biggest problem regarding the move would be that I was leaving her protective care.

We had some supper and I relayed all of the details at the radiations doctors office. I also pointed out to my mom how much I had been impressed by my new doctor. This seemed to give her some relief. "Mom, he was really very nice. I know that you will like him too."

We all decided to retire early. I knew that today had been just the beginning of a long drawn out ordeal. Unfortunately for me, I did not rest well again. My mind was concerned with what to do regarding what Brandon had offered me. I was so proud of him. He was so talented. All that work downstairs he had accomplished himself. I thought, if I sell all of the furniture that I can't use, I could use that money to help pay for all the expenses that would go along with the building of the downstairs apartment. With that in my mind, I was about to fall asleep when I remembered that I had not called Jay back. I looked at the clock and knew it was far too late to call him. "I call him first thing in the morning." I closed my eyes and fell asleep.

Okay Pam, time to get moving again. You have got to start another day. It's funny on how you never give a thought about the people that are ill. Unfortunately, I believe, as most people do, you never think that it will be you.

But it is quite a wake up call when your turn comes. I keep thinking about all the sick women in that cancer center. They all must have families. Loved ones. What a terrible thing to think that I never gave any of this a second thought until it struck home. The hospitals are full, the nursing homes are over flowing with old and lonely sick people. Oh God, please forgive me for my selfishness . I promised myself that I would learn from this experience and really try not to take everything for granted. I am going to have to train myself to be thankful for each second of the day. I know that this is not going to be easy, as this is the way I have been all my life. Shame on me.

With those last thoughts on my mind, I headed for the bathroom. Unfortunately the bleeding had started again and so had the severe pain. Can't take a pill until I eat, or I will be sick. No time to waste, just get going. Pam. I stood and maneuvered my way to the bathroom window. "Good morning world, it's Pam and I am still here. God give me strength," I said out loud." Now I don't want you to think that I just suddenly began talking to god all the time, because that is not the case. God and I had always had good relationship. No, I wasn't a big church goer, but that does not mean that I didn't believe in the Lord. I have talked to God almost every day of my life, and shall continue to do so no matter what happens.

The conversation was brief at the breakfast table. Time was at a minimum. "Mom, you don't look very good this morning. Is your heart bothering you, did you take your medicine? Please don't make me have to worry about you right now. I don't think I can handle that," I replied.

" I took my medicine, Pam. Don't worry about me," my mother answered sternly.

"Just as long as you promise that you will take care of yourself."

"I promise, she grumbled."

"Did you get any sleep, mom?"

"Oh some, I wish that I could sleep like your father. He could sleep on a picket fence. Nothing bothers him. I wish I could be like him.

I just smiled. I am sure that dad had his hearing aid shut off, which he does frequently. He confessed that one day to me, he said "it's the only way I can shut out your mother." We both laughed at that.

"I have to call Jay right now. He will be worried," I said as I headed for the living room. The phone rang about six times when a sleepy voice (Ann) answered.

"Hello?"

"Hi Ann, its Pam. I am sorry that I didn't call last night and forgive me for calling so early this morning, but I have to be in Fairfield by eight o'clock this morning. Is Jay home?

"No, you just missed him. But he will be calling me later on this morning. He was worried that he hadn't heard form you last night."

"Ann, I was so tired, forgive me. Just tell Jay that I will call him this evening. Things went well, but I will find out a lot more today. "I start my radiation treatments today, I think. But I just don't know for sure, but I will call him. Tell him I love him and kiss little Cheyenne for me, and you take care. I am okay, love you but I have to go now."

"Love you too Pam. Bye for now," and she hung up.

I put the receiver back on the phone, and turned to my mother. "Mom, are you coming with me today?"

"I don't know yet, it will depend on if Haley has gotten better and is going to school. She probably just had a bug or some schoolitis. You know how kids can be," she replied.

"I bet Rah has her dressed and ready to go to school," I said confidently. I would really like you to come today and meet Dr. Merrick. He talks in plain English not medical jargon, that you can't understand. But he does not sugar coat anything either, so be warned on what you might hear. We have got to get going, Rah will be here very shortly. So hurry and get dressed Mom."

I was right regarding Haleys sickness. Just a one day illness. Rah said, "she is fine. Come on the car is running."

On the way, my mom did her usual sputtering regarding my choice of radiation treatment centers. "Why on earth did you choose this one? The one in the Providence hospital is so much closer. It doesn't make any sense to me."

"Mom, I don't like hospitals, and unless there is no way out of going into one, I want to stay as far away from them as possible. You should be able to understand that, you hate hospitals as bad as I do. I'm telling you that you are going to like this place."

When we arrived, there were many more cars in the parking lot than yesterday. As we walked in, not many people were in the waiting area, but several employees were walking about. I started to sit in one of the chairs, when the receptionist called my name. "Ms. Ayer, please follow me."

"Can they come too, pointing to my mom and Rah?"

"That should not be a problem, as Dr. Merrick wants to see you in his office this morning before any type of treatment starts" He just wants to go over the procedures with you to try and prepare you ahead of time."

We walked into his office and he was seated behind his huge desk. Tons

75

on patients folders were scattered all around. I sat down directly in front of him and he smiled. My Mom and Rah sat over to my left in the corner of the room. "When does your first treatment of Chemotherapy start?" Dr. Merrick asked.

"Next Monday," I said.

"Well, normally, I would wait for the initial treatment of chemo to begin, but I want to proceed without any more delays. I discussed the way we are going to approach your tumor with my associate, Dr. Talbert. She agrees with me on my decision concerning how we are going to destroy this cancerous tumor. Last night, Dr. Raddison, who is a nuclear physicist, studied your biopsy. He wishes to have some special x-rays done this morning to enable him to approach the angles of radiation beams without causing any further damage to your body. This is going to be very uncomfortable for you, but unfortunately it is our only route. So, Ms. Ayer, are you ready to kill this tumor?"

"Yes, I am," I replied. "Lets get started."

"You may leave your purse with your family as it will not be needed. You need to get into the exam room and change your clothes in order for us to start this immediately!"

I gave my purse to Rah, and suggested that she and Mom take a ride and perhaps get some breakfast in the area.

"Are you sure you don't want us to stay here until you are through? We can just sit and wait."

"No, you go get at least some coffee and you can bring me back one. You two just go, I will be fine."

I followed the doctor down the hall and he pointed out the exam room where my dressing gown was waiting for me. He kept walking as I opened the door of the exam room. A nurse was unfolding a newly washed gown and placed it on table. "Please put this on and the little slippers, and when you get done just come out into the hall. "I'll be waiting for you there." I did as I was instructed (I am such a good little patient) and opened the door. Now, if you will follow me, there are a few things that I have to show you before you go to your x-rays." We walked down the hall and enter a small room filled with about a dozen lockers. The room had shelves and two small dressing rooms plus a full length mirror.

"This is where you come first before you have your radiation treatments. I am assigning you locker number nine. You needn't worry about your things as we have very good security in the building. "Once you have undressed and put on the dressing gown, you will wait in the patients waiting room until you are called. Please be on time as we usually keep our schedules right to the minute. Come with me and I will show you the patients waiting room."

We walked just a short way and walked into another doorway. "The Patients lounge." I looked in and saw a lot of people. *So that's where all the people have been, I thought.* There were men and women sitting watching tv, or reading the newspaper or a magazine. They were all dressed in johnnys. "This place is totally different from Chemo, mostly older people, especially the men. They were all older. The nurse knew them all by their first names and introduced me to each one of them. Of course, I didn't remember any of their names, but that's not unusual for me. There was such a feeling of despair in that room, I will never forget it. No smiles, no warmth. Just people sitting with no hope or future. *They can't all be dying, can they? I thought . "I won't get like that, no matter what. I wonder if depression is a side effect of radiation? Maybe that is the answer. But I won't mention it or asked any questions about it, yet.*

Another nurse met us around the next corner. "I have to get a sample of your blood and weigh you. This has to be done on a weekly basis. You must have the blood tests, or no radiation or Chemo will be administered." I made a face and she asked, "You're not afraid of needles are you?"

"Oh no, it's not the needles it's the scale I hate. I am so skinny, I don't want to know how much weight I have lost."

"Gee, I would love to have that problem, being skinny. I can't lose weight no matter how many diets I try. Guess I am destined to be fat, she sighed. Tell me how much did you normally weigh before the cancer?"

"Usually between 115-118 pounds."

"Wow, you really are a tiny one."

I stepped onto the scale and saw a horrifying sight. 95 pounds was what the scale registered. I felt sick. "Where's the bathroom, I am going to be sick."

"Right down the hall, first door on the left, it has a sign on it." Believe me when I say, I just about made it. I gagged and finally lost what breakfast I had in my stomach. *Be strong, be strong.* I splashed some water on my face and stayed in there until I could regain myself.

There was a tapping on the door. "Are you alright, do you need the doctor?"

"I am okay. I will be right out," I replied weakly.

When I stepped out of the bathroom, the two nurses were waiting for me. "Do you need help walking?"

"No, I am okay now. Once it comes up, I feel better, thank you. I just got upset when I saw how skinny I actually am."

The last room that I was brought into was very similar to an operating room.

It had lots of ceiling lights and instruments. There was a huge overhead machine, which I have never see the likes of anywhere, and of course the table in the middle of the floor with stirrups. I was instructed to get onto the table and lie back. One of the nurses came over and pulled up my dressing gown revealing my "*Victoria Secrets*" panties. She took a Polaroid camera off the counter and began to take pictures. She took pictures of each and every part of my lower body. I was never so embarrassed in my life.

"I am sorry, and I know this is difficult for you, but these are needed as a type of body map for the radiation beams," the nurse confessed. If that wasn't degrading enough, next came some white stuff forced into my rectum, and then a spectrum was placed in my vagina with more of the white stuff. The nurses left the room and instructed me to lie perfectly still. The machine began to move making ungodly sounds. I was terrified, humiliated, and ready to scream. The machine began to slow down and I knew that it was almost over. I lay there as still as a statue. Not wanting to disturb anything that was in my body. I was afraid that if I did, they would have to repeat the process.

It was over, the machine was painless, but not my shame. My pride was gone. Any type of shyness that I had ever had disappeared that morning. I started to cry. No, not cry, sob. My tears were uncontrollable. I just couldn't stop. The nurse came over and gave me some tissues and at that moment Dr. Merrick walked in. He walked over to me and took my hand. "It's okay, it's just the reality of it all sinking in. Let it all out and you will feel better. It's perfectly normal to feel what you are feeling." It was at that moment I realized that Dr. Merrick was a true gentleman. He truly cared about how I felt. I was a real person, not just another patient to him. He pulled my gown back down to its proper position and instructed the nurses to give me a minute or two. He smiled at me and left the room.

"Do you need anything, Ms. Ayer?" another nurse asked.

I managed to get a weak, "No," out of my mouth."

"You may remain here until you feel that you are up to moving. Then you can go and get dressed. Just call out, if you need anyone ."

I was so ashamed that I had lost it in front of all those strangers. I just had totally lost control. I can't swear to it, but I don't believe that I cried again in front of anyone again during my illness. I stayed there for a few more minutes, and then weakly swung my legs over to the side of the table and got my feet on the floor. What's that phrase? "Come on feet, don't fail me now," was all I could think about. I shuffled all the way into the bathroom and stuffed all sorts of paper towels into my underwear. I just wanted to make sure that I could get to the locker room without leaking whatever they put into me all over the floor. That is one embarrassment that I could not of tolerated at that moment. I got dressed and walked into the hallway, sort of hoping that Rah and Mom would not be there yet, but there they were, waiting for me.

The nurse who had taken the Polaroids smiled and said, "I'll see you tomorrow." I hoped that neither Rah or my mom could tell by my face that I had been crying.

When we got to the car it was only 9:30 in the morning and I was already exhausted.

"Do you need something to eat, Mom?" Rah asked.

"No, let's just go home. I really feel awful."

"Should I ask what happened?"

"No, let's just forget it for now. I'll tell you someday. But I will tell you this, I think today was probably the worst day I have had so far. I know that I have many more to come, but I don't think that they can top today."

"I was thinking Mom, Rah said suddenly, Why don't you come over to my house for supper? You can rest all afternoon. The kids are in school, and you can lay down on my bed and sleep."

"Yes, I think I will do just that." I looked at my mother and said,"Mom, you and Dad go play your card games with your friends. You will be home in plenty of time. You know how much Dad enjoys playing "Hi Low Jack." There is no reason for you two not to go."

"Well, are you sure, Pam?" my mom asked.

"Yes, definitely. Besides, it will give me a chance to see the kids. My mom agreed reluctantly and we dropped her off. But before she got into the house, she turned and came back to the car. "Make sure your home in plenty of time to get your sleep tonight."

"Yes mother dear." I smiled at her, and we drove away.

Chapter 20
The Kids

Rah lives about a mile from my parents apartment. She lives in a large house that is in need of a lot of repair. But financially she and her family are pretty strapped, and have to settle for this house for the time being. The house is large enough for the four kids and Rah and her husband, plus the rent is reasonable. So right now, this is where they have to remain. It's a nice neighborhood for the kids and the school system is very good.

Having lived in Rhode Island my entire life, I can tell you first hand that houses are very expensive. But when you have four kids (and another baby on the way) finding one that is big enough, and nice inside, plus fits your price range, is extremely difficult. In better times, I could have helped them with the money they need. But not now and that makes me feel totally helpless, no, worthless describes it better. I should be in a position to help my family, not take from them.

When we arrived at Rah's, I went inside and asked if I could use her bedroom to lie down in for a short time?

"Mom, that is why I brought you here. How much rest do you actually get on Nana's couch?" I know that she wanted to talk, but I needed to clear my head and try and catch up on my sleep while I had the opportunity. Escaping reality is so easy when you sleep. So I made my escape to her bedroom and slept.

It was dusk when I opened my eyes, and I could feel someone starring at me even though I was not totally awake. I turned over and saw three little faces, all smiles, just standing there grinning at me. The tallest and next to the oldest is Tawnee. She is her mothers clone. Thin, long red hair, freckles and a turned up nose. She looks so much like her mother when Rah was a child, just looking at her brings me back in time to my little girl Robin. Next in line was Haley. Another redhead, but chubbier than her older sister. She had beautiful blue eyes and a bubbling personality. Her smile was never ending. She was always happy. Last but by no means least was the one and only Kyle (name). He was the only boy in any of the families. Which of course means he is special. He has dark brown hair and big brown eyes. I think Kyle (name) looked the most like me of all my grandchildren. I hate to say it, but I think that he is going to have my nose. Now let me explain about the Kyle (name) business. When he was only a toddler, about 2 or 3, when someone asked him his name, he would reply "Kyle name." Now, three years later, he is still known as Kyle name. Someday I know that he will lose the word "name," but I kind of hope that it is not too soon. I like it, and it always makes me laugh.

"Hi Meme," they all yelled at the same time. Mommy has got supper ready. She told Daddy that you have slept all day."

"She did, did she? Well, you know what? She was right. I was a very sleepy Meme. I am glad that you awakened me."

"Tawnee walked up closer to me and asked, "Meme, we heard Mommy and Daddy talking and they said that you have cancer."

"Do you have cancer? Cancer is bad isn't it?"

"Well Miss Tawnelda (another nickname), I do have cancer, but I am hoping that it is not the real bad cancer. The doctors are going to try and kill all of the cancer in my body, so that I can be healthy again. Do you understand?"

Haley spoke up, "I do, I know that you will get better soon. Right Meme?"

"Right!" Do you have anything you want to ask me Kyle (name)?

"Yes, do you want to eat now, because I am hungry?"

I laughed and teased him and said " I hope your mommy didn't make her speciality, hotdogs."

A voice from the kitchen said, "I heard that. No, it's not hot dogs! I prepared two different suppers. I didn't know which one you would be in the mood for, so I made baked chicken or if you prefer home made beef stew. Which would you like?"

"I'll take some of both." The kids all laughed. Now if you little ones can pull me up out of this bed, I will go to the supper table." The three of them all charged me at the same time. But surprisingly they were very, very gentle.

They headed me for the living room, where am I going?"

"Mommy said that you were going to eat in the living room."

"Well, I better not argue with her, cause she is tough."

Greg was standing in the kitchen helping Rah, and said, "Well look who is finally awake."

"Yea, I just about remember laying down. Do I look like sleeping beauty, or the evil queen?' Never mind, don't answer that. "

" I'll bring supper to you Mom, which one of them do you want?"

"Oh, I want to sit at the table with all of you. Now don't argue with me Rah, I am still your mother and I am going to eat the table."

The supper was excellent. The kids were delightful. Kyle (name) had macaroni and cheese. This is his all time favorite. Rah and Greg have found it easier to give him what he wants rather than to listen to him complain. He is one of those little treasures that gags when you try to make him eat something he doesn't want.

After supper I was promptly sent to the couch. "Greg and I will do the dishes, Mom. The kids want you to play Nintendo with them. They have a new game called "Super Mario." We had just began playing the game, when I heard the phone ring. Tawnee brought it over to me, "I's uncle Jay."

"Hi mom. How did it go today? What's happening and why are you at Rah's?"

"It went okay at the doctors, and I am doing alright. I am at Rah's just to get away from my mom for a little while. She is so worried about me, that I am afraid that she will have another heart attack. So Rah asked me to come for supper, and I took her up on it. How's things with you and your family?"

"Dad called today."

"Oh, what did he want?"

"He just asked how you were doing and wanted to know if you were still living in the house? He said that he will give you ten thousand dollars for it, if you sign the deed over to him. That way you won't have to lose it to the bank."

"Well isn't that kind of him. A whole ten thousand dollars. He knows the house is worth at least one hundred and fifty thousand dollars. What a jerk! Jay, you tell him that I will gladly lose the house to the bank any day than to ever let him have it. Over my dead body. That's a bad way of putting it. Your father will never get that house from me.

"I am sorry Mom, I didn't want to upset you, but you know how he is. He is going to be calling me back shortly."

"Just give him my message."

"Is there anything that Ann and I can do?"

"Not unless you have tons of money hidden somewhere."

"I am afraid that we are all in the same sinking boat," Jay replied.

"You just take care of your family son, and I will call you and keep you posted on what is going on. Love you and thanks for calling."

Oh the nerve of that man. Please God, don't let me have hate in my heart. Forgiveness, Pam remember forgiveness. Don't think about it anymore. Remember he is a sick man.

While Greg and Rah worked in the kitchen, the kids and I started to play Nintendo. "You have to sit on the floor, Meme," Haley said.

"Okay, I'll try." We all sat down in front of the tv and Tawnee turned on the machine. It was the cutest game. Very interesting. The kids made it look easy that is until I tried to do it. Haley was laughing so hard.

"I can't do it, I yelled. What am I doing wrong?"

"Oh you just need practice. You'll get so you do can do it Meme, don't worry, Tawnee said smiling." It is amazing how easily children can handle these games. Adults are all thumbs. We continued laughing and played for almost an hour. My pain was returning and I told the children that I had to quit for a little while and rest.

"Leave Meme alone now kids. Go on outside and play for a while." Tawnee shut off the game with a little mumbling under her breath. She hugged me and headed out the door with her brother and sister. Rah and Greg came into the living room and sat down one on each side of me. Oh boy, here comes the talk, I thought. I can see it coming.

Rah started first. " Mom, have you thought about Brandon's offer?"

Greg interrupted with, "I think it is much better for you than staying at your mothers."

Well, I really haven't had much of a chance to think about it yet, but my first reaction to it is very favorable. I really appreciate all that you kids are doing for me."

"Mom, we all love you. It's our turn now, let us help. Let Brandon help."

"I realize what you are all trying to do. Just let me think about it for a few days. I's a big decision and it affects a lot of peoples lives, not just mine."

Rah, would you get me a pain pill out of my purse? I have to go to the bathroom again. I wish I could keep some food in me for at least four or five hours. But no, here I go again. Please remind me to ask one of the doctors for some medicine to help me with this. There has to be something I can take that will stop it. I can't keep losing weight. I am getting weaker every day."

When I returned from the bathroom, I knew that I should be going back to

83

my mom's house. She would be calling and having a fit. Before I left, I hugged the kids and told them to behave themselves. They promised they would. "You can call me anytime, kids, you know where I am. Love you, bye."

"Love you too Meme." I waved and smiled, and once again, I was on the move.

Once we were on our way, I asked Rah, "Where is little Miss Amanda?

"Oh she is with her girlfriends today. Or at least that is where she said she was going. I don't know what I am going to do with her?"

"How is she feeling?"

"The doctor said she is fine and so is the baby. She shouldn't have any problems even though she is so young, if she is careful."

It had only been a couple of weeks since we found out she was pregnant. I know there are much worse things in this world than having a child, but a child having a child is another story.

" I don't want to think about it, I told Rah. It breaks my heart."

"Mom, I am trying so hard to be strong, but I am not like you."

"You can handle anything, Mom," Rah replied.

"Rah, you had Amanda when you were seventeen. You of all people should know what she is going through. She is going to need you."

"But Amanda is so difficult, mom. She tells me stories all the time, and I know that she is still seeing that boy."

"It will pass, the boy will loose interest as soon as she starts getting fat. Right now, its romantic. Their just kids. But I want you to remember this, you're my daughter and you can handle it. Just keep telling yourself that. I have faith in you."

We parked in front of my parents apartment, and she reached for the door handle. "Don't bother Ra, I can make it easily. See you in the morning. I Love you, and I leaned over and kissed her. "Bye, daughter dear, I opened the door and when I got to the door of the apartment, I gave her the signal that all was fine and she drove away.

Both of my parents were up when I came in the door. "What did you eat? Did you keep it down? I hope those kids didn't tire you out."

"Rah cooked a wonderful meal, and I enjoyed it very much. As of this very minute, so far I have kept it in me (lying again). The kids were great. We just sat around playing their new Nintendo game."

"Did you see Amanda?"

"No, she wasn't home, but Rah said she was with her girlfriends. But I suspect that she was most likely with her boyfriend. She has no idea of how much her life is going to change when that baby arrives. Peter is only sixteen years old. How on earth is he going to pay for a child? My mother just shook her head. I suggested to Rah that she take Amanda down to the Welfare office and see if they can assist in any way. I know that Amanda is covered on Greg's medical, but I don't know about if they will cover the baby once he is born.

" Well I think the whole thing is crazy, my Mom said. She should give the baby up for adoption."

"Your probably right Mom, but she never will do it. Can we discuss something else? I just can't think about it anymore right now. I'll just think about it tomorrow."

"Did you and Dad win at your card game today?"

"We won five out of seven games, Dad replied. That puts us in second place and if we win, we will get $100. That would help out a lot right now."

Guilt trip, on my part, after hearing that. I know that it is costing them money by me staying here. I couldn't help but think, if she thinks she is broke, she should see my bank account. Zip, zero, zilch. Why does she think I am losing my house? Don't think about it now. You had a nice evening with your grand children. I will worry about the cancer, and Amanda, and money tomorrow.

I was not looking forward to tomorrow. At least it's Friday and maybe there will be a chance that treatments were not done on the weekend. I had that thought to keep me going. I really didn't sleep much, but I used the night to think. I am going to have to make a decision soon. Brandon had already done so much work what harm would it be to try it. I will call him and tell him about my thoughts regarding the sale of all my furniture. My furniture was not that old and in good shape. I will just put it in the paper and let the kids handle the people and the sales.

I lay there thinking, *I will have to have Brandon put in a bathroom right away. The bathroom was just to far away for me. Especially with my stomach problems. That was my last thought for the night.*

Chapter 21
Tattoos

Another morning of rushing around. God I was sick. Rah arrived at 7:30. She looked as tired as I felt. I looked at my mom and said, "Come on Mom, it's another beautiful day in the HUD neighborhood. Let me grab my sweater." Rah laughed out loud. But our little private joke went right over my moms head, which only made us laugh that much more. So we headed for the car wearing smiles.

Once I arrived at the doctors office, I immediately walked the corridor to the locker room. Rah and Mom were going over to Susan's house while I was getting my first treatment. I could see that staying at Brandon's house would be a great advantage. Poor Rah would not have to get up so early and get the kids ready for school. The worse part was that the kids school bus did not come until almost nine o'clock. That meant that the children were alone for almost an hour and a half. Dad offered to go up and sit with them, but right now he was having car problems. Thankfully Rah's neighbor offered to watch the kids every day for us until dads' car was fixed.

I hung up my clothes and put my purse in locker number nine, took a quick look in the mirror, and just shook my hear with disgust and continued on my way. Next stop the "Patients Lounge." The patients were all there. Same as yesterday, just sitting there, no conversations, just blank stares. "Good morning everyone," I said while sitting down in the only empty chair. A few of them did look up and acknowledge my greeting. I could almost read their minds. What has she got to be so happy about? Wait until she does this for months, she will change her attitude. I knew in my heart that they were wrong. I was going to face this with positive thoughts, no matter what they did to me. I studied the patients, scanning each and every one of them with my eyes. Some of them were wearing their dressing gowns with trousers on, while others wore their gowns without trousers. I was not wearing trousers. I quickly came to the brilliant conclusion that some of the patients had upper body cancer, while others had cancer in the lower part of their bodies. The man to my left was reading the newspaper. He never looked up. But the woman to my right actually said "would you please pass the Newsweek magazine to me."

I smiled at her and replied, "Sure."

"Your new. I saw you yesterday."

"Yes, I am here for my very first treatment."

"Well, young lady, I wish you luck."

"I have breast cancer and have been through this before. It's not much fun. Perhaps you will be one of the lucky ones."

"I plan on it, I said firmly."

"Good, you're a fighter, and honey that is what you need to be."

"Mrs. Peterson, we are ready for you."

"That's me. Bye honey." She left the room with the nurse. She was not dressed like me, she had trousers on. I wouldn't even try and guess her age. Her sickness had taken it's toll. That was very plain to see. A few minutes passed and then it was my turn. As I was leaving the Patients Lounge, I saw them bringing in a very elderly woman in on a stretcher. The nurse read my mind and commented,"She is a patient from the hospital across the street. We have a number of patients brought in and also other patients from the nursing home down the street. They are brought in by ambulance for their treatments."

"Before we start your treatment today, we have to get a blood sample and weigh you. Then it's back into the same room that you were in yesterday. Today is Tattoo Day."

"Oh my word" was all I could say."

"Well, it's not what you think. The tattoos are very small, similar to a freckle. It's like playing connect the dots. They follow the dots with the radiation beams."

Once in the room, I was assisted in getting onto the table. "This won't hurt, just little pin pricks." At that moment, Dr. Merrick came into the room carrying large manilla envelopes. I presume they were my x-rays from yesterday. He placed them on a lighted screen on the wall.

"Well, Ms Ayer, are you ready to get your tattoos?

87

"Yes I am doctor. I already have one on my ankle."

"I noticed that one. When did you get that?" Dr. Merrick replied.

"About two years ago, it was to celebrate my divorce. It's a replica of my favorite stamp and my favorite flower. A beautiful yellow rose."

He smiled, and said, "It's very becoming on you."

"Thank you doctor."

"Please do not move when they are measuring you. This is very important. Stay perfectly still."

"I won't move doctor," I assured him. There were three nurses, Dr. Merrick and another man in the room with me. I did not recognize the other man. Everyone was very serious and extremely quiet. No one made a sound. The calculations were done, (I don't have the slightest idea how) and the areas were then marked with a black marker. Every mark was checked, measured, and checked again. Finally I felt the pin pricks. I think I ended up with eight or nine new freckles. They were placed in different locations on my lower body.

"That does it. You can go into room #3 for your first treatment Ms. Ayer. I will see you later on. Good luck," and the doctor left the room. I squirmed my way to the edge of the table, swung my legs over the side and stood up.

"Treatment room # 3 is down the corridor just a short ways on your right. Do need any assistance walking?"

"No, I can manage. I can find it." The room was only a short walk away and when I entered into it, there were two nurses waiting for me.

"Come right up here, young lady, patting the exam table. This won't take anytime at all. It will be over in a heart beat. So don't look so nervous. We won't hurt you a bit." She was smiling all the time she was talking to me."

I slowly positioned myself on the table. What they were doing, I couldn't tell you. I was just too busy checking out this new machine. It wasn't as massive as the last one I had been introduced to, but it was very impressive looking. The two nurses (or assistants, I am never sure) were busy taking some kind of blocks and placing them around the table. I am just not sure if the blocks were a type of guideline or if they were films of some sort. But I do know that they had my name on them. I truly can't remember things very clearly whether that is caused by a mental block on my part or the medication, I can't say.

"Now we have to leave the room, Ms. Ayer. Please do not move. The machine will do all the moving. It will encircle your body. Remember, don't move until you hear me give you the go a head."

"Okay, I understand." I don't know exactly what I expected, but I felt nothing. The machine hummed, whirred, and continually moved, but I felt absolutely nothing. It only last for a few short moments.

"Okay, all clear. You can move now, we are coming back in."

"I'm done? That's it?" The two ladies were both back in the room.

"Yep that is it for today. How do you feel?"

"Fine."

" Well, that's good. We'll see you again soon." They both began removing the blocks from around the table and filed them in a spot built into the wall with my name printed on it. I got up off the table and said my goodbyes and left the room.

Boy was I glad that was over. I returned to the locker room, changed and went to the front reception desk. "May I use the phone?"

"Of course, she said.

I called Susan's house, and Sue answered right away.

"Hello?" She said.

"I am all done, Sue. Can you send Rah to come and pick me up?" She is grabbing her coat right now. Are you up for a visit?"

"No, I would really rather go home right now. But thanks. I'll call you later, okay?"

"Sure Pam, you go home and rest."

I hung up the phone and thanked the receptionist. "Well we will see again Monday morning then, Ms. Ayer?"

"Oh no, I can't. I have to be in Providence for Chemo first thing Monday morning."

"Alright, then just come here right after your Chemo. I will schedule you for around two o'clock. That should give you enough time to get here from Providence."

As I sat there waiting for Rah and my mother, my mind was consumed by questions. I know that I should ask questions regarding the treatments, a lot of questions, but I never could bring myself to question anything the doctors did. Perhaps I can blame my lack of asking questions because I really didn't want to know what they were doing to me, I was frightened of hearing something that would terrify me even more than I was. Or maybe it was the medication I was taking. But somewhere inside me, I believe it is called blind faith or trust. Who was I to question a doctor?

I saw Rah pull in the parking lot, and I was out the door before she could park her car. I noticed as we were driving home, everyone was very quiet. I couldn't help but wonder if some type of argument had taken place between my mother and Susan. I really hoped that Sue and Rah had stayed away from the newly installed bedroom issue. My Mom would get really upset if she heard the news from Susan and not me. I know that I am a grown woman but having my Mom angry with me is still very upsetting. Silly, isn't? But it turned out that Rah and my mom were just worried about what the radiation would do to me, and what kind of condition I would be in when they picked me up. I tried to sooth their worries and explained to them that it had been almost totally painless. Other than the pin pricks, their had been no additional pain that day. *As we drove along, all I could think tomorrow is Saturday. I really need a break. A couple of days without the stress of all these new treatments and I will feel a lot better. I would really enjoy going somewhere. Just a nice ride in the country. It's fall right now and the leaves are beautiful. I have always loved the fall season. But riding would prove to be difficult with my bathroom problems and my pain.* "Shit," I said out loud.

"What" both Rah and my mother echoed. "I forgot to ask Dr. Merrick for some stomach medicine. Please Rah don't let me forget to mention some medication when we go to the Chemo center."

"I'll remind you, don't worry."

"Write it down," my mother advised.

"I will, Mom and you write it down too Rah. That way we both will have reminders."

Rah drove up to my moms apartment and asked, "Anything you need?"

"No, but thanks. You go home and tend to your family. Once again Rah, thank you."

"Stop worrying about me, Mom" and take care of yourself."

"Tell the kids I said hello."

"I will, I'll call you later and check in with you."

Mom walked in the apartment and said to dad before we could even get our coats off, "Pam got tattoos today at the treatment center. Can you imagine that?"

"Your kidding, real tattoos?"

"Oh Dad, not like you think. Their tiny like little freckles." Then I began to explained, to the best of my ability the plan of Dr. Merrick. How each radiation beam followed the placements of the tattooed dots. Dad seemed to grasp what I was trying to explain; however my mother on the other hand, was definitely lost. It was either that or she just didn't want to understand. Sometimes she had the tendency to understand only what she wanted to accept.

The subject was changed, and Mom moved on to Susan. "Well, I must say Susan has really decorated her house very nicely. I wonder how they can afford all that fancy furniture?"

"Mom, Sue and Brandon do not have a lot of money. Brandon works his tail off, and he lets Susan buy what she wants. I know for a fact the furniture looks a great deal more expensive that it really costs. She loves nice things. It's just the way she is. When you were young Mom, didn't you spend money on what you wanted? Plus, she keeps those girls looking just like models. Give her some credit, all the money does not go for just what she wants."

I sat there listening to my mother go on and on and thought to myself, boy Mom, are you going to be mad when you hear what Brandon has done regarding my new bedroom. But you will get over it, because you love me. Tomorrow I am going to have to go over to Rah's house and call Brandon. It's for sure that I can't talk to him here. There is just no way for me to please everybody. At least I know Rah will be okay with it, but Jason is going to be another story. He won't like the idea that I will be giving my money to his brother, and he won't look at it in the proper light. He will only see that Brandon is getting money from me. I have helped both Rah and Jason with money before. Brandon has never asked me for much, and I truly believe that he is doing this to help me, not improve the value of his house. I will just have to do what I think is best for me this time.

I sat there and thought about how I was going to approach this matter regarding the sale of my furniture, and I have got to write out a "Will" as well. If I should die, I want it all in writing so there can be no fighting among my children. I already have a life insurance policy through the post office leaving all the money to my three children, and it shall be divided equally among them, so no one thinks one received more than the other. I really won't have much after I sell everything, but what is left will go to the three of them. That was one thing that I did when I was married about which my ex had no knowledge. When I bought the policy, my ex thought he was going to be the beneficiary. The joke was on him. His name was never there. Only the children. He will never get one dime from my death. Not one dime. That thought made me smile.

I spent the rest of the day on the couch. Just dozing on and off in between conversations with my Mom and Dad. It must have been around six or seven when the door bell rang. "Who could that be, I said? Maybe it's Ra?"

"No it's Jay with Ann and the baby," my mom answered as she was looking out the window. "Open the door and let them in. Hi, what a nice surprise," I said happily.

Jay leaned over and gave me a quick kiss. "Hi Mom. We just wanted to come over and see you. Sorry it's so of late. We had to stop in and check in on my mother, and she lives so close to you, we thought you wouldn't mind if we just said hello and stayed a few minutes.

"How are you doing Pam?" Ann asked.

"Really pretty good Ann. I have great confidence in the doctors." She was holding little Cheyenne in her arms. Little Cheyenne was asleep, but absolutely adorable. I touched her little hand and gave it a little squeeze.

Ann sat down next to me and asked, "What happened today?"

"Well, I got some tattoos and had my first radiation treatment. My radiation doctor, Dr. Merrick, seems to be very positive in regards to getting all of this tumor of mine. The chemo doctor, Dr. Johnson, doesn't say much except, Ms. Ayer, you are going to lose all of your hair. I was thinking about that Ann, what do you think? Should I shave all my hair off now, or wait and let it fall out in clumps?"

It was at that moment that my son got up and walked into the kitchen. I could hear him crying. "Oh God, he is so tender hearted, what am I going to do with him?" Jay had totally lost it. I heard a chair go flying. Mom and dad jumped up and headed for the kitchen. I held on to Ann and shook my head and said "NO," to her. Let him alone Ann. It will pass."

"But Pam, he has been like this since we got the news about the cancer."

"I know, it's hard for him to accept. Be patient with him, please Ann."

We could hear the conversation very clearly that was taking place in the kitchen. My Mom yelled, "Stop it right now and get a hold of yourself."

"Dad simply said, "Now is not the time."

Jay's answer was plain and loud. "Well, it should be Dad, not Mom! He is the one that should bet sick. Not Mom, she never hurt anyone, and he hurts everyone.

My father spoke again, "Jay your mother needs you to be strong, so I suggest that you stop this right now."

It was so hard for me to sit there. I wanted to run to my son and comfort him like I had so many times before when he was a little child. His father had always favored Brandon. Poor Jay could never do anything to his fathers satisfaction. And Jay always tried so hard. My ex considered Jay to be weak. Maybe Jay was weak in a way, but I call it a gentleness that most men don't have. Jay was never cold hearted and hateful. Jay had pity for everything, especially animals, even a Lassie movie could make Jay cry when he was a boy. That would infuriate his father. "You have to be a man."

"Men don't cry." But Jay had grown up to be a man, a good man despite his fathers negative influence. But the damage that his father had managed to

CRYING IN THE SHOWER - CERVICAL CANCER

inflict was very visible especially to me. Why had I stayed in a marriage with a man who was destroying my son? I still ask God every day to forgive me for my selfishness. After a few more words by my parents, there was silence in the kitchen. I heard the chair being moved once again. Then total silence. Dad went into his room and Mom came back into the living room.

Jay sat in the kitchen for a while and gathered his emotions. I know that he was having difficulty in returning to the living room to face me because he was embarrassed and ashamed of his outburst. I yelled out to him, "Jay, would you get me a drink of soda please?"

"Sure Mom," his voice was shaky. A few more moments passed and in came Jay with my soda.

"Thanks Jay."

"Your welcome, Mom." Nothing else was said about my illness that evening. I wasn't going to go there again, and I stayed away from the subject entirely.

"So how is work going Jay?"

"Not that great right now. The weather has been too rainy to do much cement work."

Jay had tried just about every type of work that a man could do outside. He loved the outdoors. He was an extremely hard worker but never seemed to get that "break" that he deserved. He totally enjoyed working with his hands outdoors. It didn't matter whether it was tree work, yard work, or cement work. Just as long as he was in the fresh air he was happy, and how he loved fishing and hunting.

I wish that Jay had chosen to go to college so that he could have been a Park Ranger or something on that line. He had been graduated with honors. Not so with his brother or his sister. Not that Jay wasn't popular, because he was. He was as handsome as a boy could be, but he didn't want to settle down with one girl. Brandon fell in love with Susan (his first girlfriend) and Rah became pregnant when she was seventeen. School was not that interesting to them. Friends and fun meant more to them then studying. But Jay tried hard, always trying to please his father and to make his father notice him. But I can't think about this right now, maybe tomorrow.

"Mom, what are you doing this weekend? Are you up to anything?"

"Well, I don't know Jay. "I feel okay right now, and I don't have anything planned. Why? If you feel up to it, would you like us to pick you up and bring you to our house for Sunday dinner? I'll have you home in plenty of time so that you can rest for Monday.

That's a very nice invitation, Jay. I would enjoy that very much. Sounds like a date, then."

"Sunday it is, Mom." They stayed and visited for about another hour. Cheyenne never woke up during the entire visit. Poor little pumpkin, she must have been really tired. So we said our good byes and hugged each other, but carefully.

"Call me tomorrow, Ann."

"Oh I will, you take it easy. Drive carefully. Bye"

Chapter 22

Saturday

Surprise, I got a great nights sleep last night. Maybe the radiation will make me tired enough to sleep. Maybe that's its side effect. I smiled at that thought. Like I am going to get that lucky? Dad had already left to go to the drug store and purchase some over the counter medicine for my bathroom problem. But at least last night the diarrhea did not interrupt my sleep. I have to be very careful what I put in my stomach. My biggest problem is I love coffee. Especially that first cup in the morning. I know that it is definitely not good for me, but I can't seem to function without it. Plus I get crabby if I don't get it and everyone in the family knows it. It is about the only time, that you will catch me in a terrible mood. I don't think I could give up my coffee even if both doctors told me too. True, I had received two separate diet instructions (one from each doctor) and each diet listed what I should be eating, not what I couldn't have. So for now, I was safe with my morning coffee.

Today should be an interesting day. First on the list was to get myself to Rah' house to enable me to call Brandon without my mother knowing what was going on. I have to tell him about my idea regarding the sale of the furniture. I am sure he will agree to the idea, plus I must get moving on this. The clock is ticking. Things have to be arranged before I get too sick to do anything, and I want to be there when the furniture is sold. I know what it is worth better than anyone else, therefore I must insist on this, no matter what the kids have to say about it.

Around eleven, Rah called. "Hi Mom, any side effects from the first radiation treatment?"

"No Rah, if there were any, I slept right through them."

"That's a relief. I was afraid that you would be sick, I was really worried about you."

"Rah, we have just stepped up to the first level of getting rid of this tumor."

"Very true Ma."

"Are you coming after me, or do you want me to get Dad to drive me up to your house?"

"It really doesn't matter Mom, whatever?"

"Well, I just got up and I am not even dressed yet."

"Me either, Rah replied.

"I'll just ask dad drive me up to your house after I get dressed. I'll see you shortly. Tell the kids to turn on the Nintendo."

"Don't worry Ma, they already have it on. They're waiting for you."

"Tell them that I will be there in a few minutes."

"Okay, see you in a few."

After the conversation was finished, I told my Mom about my plans for the day. "I really wish that you would stay home today and just rest. You know you have to keep up your strength with every thing that you are going to be facing. I think that you are over doing with all the company and you planning to visit Rah today and Jay tomorrow."

"I know, I know but I am trying to get some living in before I reach the point of not being able to do anything at all."

"Well for the record, I definitely don't think that you should travel all the way to Jay's house tomorrow."

"Mom, these are my kids and only God knows if I am going to have a lot more time left with any of them. Besides mom, I know how they are. Once I start getting worse from the treatments or if something unforseen happens and they find more cancer, my kids are not going to handle it well at all. I plan on spending all the time I can with them right now, while I can. Call me crazy, but there is a method to my madness. I also need to be around you, and I need you too Mom. But I don't want to jeopardize your health by you worrying about me all the time either. No matter what happens or where I am, you are my mother and I will always need you. But for now, please let me do things my way when it comes to my kids."

"Alright, but I don't have to agree with you. Just remember you're the one who is sick. You should be looking out for yourself instead of worrying about how your children are going to handle things."

"Seeing my children and being with them makes me feel better. Being around the grand children gives me strength and a reason to get better. It gives me something to live for, and my life has been so bad lately, that it's a rare feeling to be happy. My family give me what I need, mom, so please try and understand my feelings."

After the conversation, I headed for the bathroom. My private crying place. The most important thing I discovered about the bathroom is the shower.... it is the best place to cry. I think a lot of women know about this secret, but I have just recently discovered it. I can cry in the shower and nobody knows or would even suspect. If someone asks about why my eyes are red, I just say, some of the soap from the shampoo must have gotten into them. It's a wonderful place to let all your feelings out. Most people sing in the shower, I cry. All my secret thoughts and heart aches are safe in the secret crying place know only as the shower.

It was little Haley that opened the door when I arrived at the house. Her usual big smile greeted me. "Come on in, Meme we have been waiting for you. The game is all set up."

I walked in and Tawnee and Kyle (name) were already on the floor playing the game. Amanda was on the couch with her usual glass of milk in one hand and a bag of potato chips in the other. "Hi Meme" she said without moving from her prone position. "How are you feeling?"

"I'm good, and you?"

"Oh, I am still sick every morning. When does it stop?"

"My dear, you have a long way to go. Morning sickness usually last about the three or four months of the pregnancy, but you can ask the doctor to give you something that will ease it a bit. I found that eating dry crackers, first thing in the morning, will help relieve the nausea."

"Come over and sit with me, Meme." She sat up and motioned for me to come over to her. "Kyle (name) is doing pretty good. He has already reached the third level of the game."

"Boy that is good! I can't even last a minute without getting myself killed." Kyle (name) stopped and turned around and gave me a winning smile and then quickly continued playing. He was totally consumed by the game. What I find so unusual about the way he plays it is, he cannot sit down and play. He has to stand and is in constant motion. He moves with the character on the tv screen. He twists left and right and jumps up and down constantly.

"Come on Kyle, give me a turn," Haley asked.

"Wait a minute, wait a minute," Kyle (name) shouted.

Rag was standing in the kitchen window, trying to put on some make-up, when she spoke up. "No arguing, or the game gets shut off. Kyle, give your sister a turn right now."

Amanda turned her attention from the game to me. "So Meme, tell me all about the doctors?" "There is not an awful lot to tell yet, but I am planning to be around when my first great grand child enters this world." I had been blessed, I had seen the birth of all my grand children. Each and every one of them. My children had requested that I be present for the delivery of each child. I was usually the first one to touch the newborn and to hold each and everyone right after they were born. How lucky is that? I don't think that there are that many grandmothers in this world who has had the honor of seeing seven grandchildren born. Now at the age of 54, I am going to be a great grandmother. "I have no intention of missing your babies birth. Of course you know that it will be a boy."

"Any chance that you might be wrong Meme? I really want a little girl."

"Nope, I haven't been wrong yet little girl, and I am positive that you are carrying a son. So don't buy pink." Amanda snuggled up close to me. I thought to myself, how can this child become a mother? She was such a little girl herself. It broke my heart. Poor Amanda, she was such a mixed up girl. She had always craved the attention of her mother, but Rah was too young herself to be a mother. And so the circle repeats itself. Amanda will make the same mistakes her mother made and all my advise will not change anything. "God, life is so strange."

"I pray that I will be around to see my grand children grow up. Even though heart aches and head aches come with each one of them, I want to be here to see it. "Not my will, but thy will." Please Lord, give me strength,

Sometimes it takes all I have inside me, not to scream. I can't be sick, I want to live. My children and grandchildren need me. I want the chance to do all the things that I used to dream about. A real nice vacation, meeting someone who thinks I am special. A new beginning. I don't want to grow old alone, and the thought of that scared me more than cancer. Maybe this is Gods way of seeing to it that I don't have to grow old alone. Maybe it's his way of saving me from that pain. I could kick myself for all the time I wasted on such a cold cruel man. Cry in the shower, Pam, and think about it tomorrow.

Rah came in from the kitchen and looked at the crazy crew in the living room. They we were, Amanda with her head on my shoulder, Tawnee on the other side of me with her arm around me and Haley at my feet. Of course, Kyle (name) was still playing the game. "Well, this is a picture."

"Can you get any closer to Meme? How about letting her have some breathing room?"

"Oh their fine, Rah. My don't you look pretty, Rah."

"You think? It only took me an hour to fix my make up and my hair."

"I told you, the older you get the longer it takes to look good." We both chuckled at that one. But we also knew it was a true statement.

"I thought we might go for a little ride, if your up to it, Mom?"

"I really need to go to my home Rah, and get some clothes."

"Do you think you should do that Mom? You know how it is going to upset you."

"No, don't worry, I have got a handle on it this morning. I have resigned myself to the fact I am losing the house, and the house takes last place about things to worry about right now. It's too late to save the old homestead. Besides there is so much to be packed and cleaned. I can't keep putting it off. I haven't been home in days. I just hope that nothing has happened, like your father breaking in and taking stuff."

"I am sure that it is fine, Mom. Besides the neighbors would be watching it."

"Well they would if I asked them to, but they don't know what has happened."

"I am sure that they have noticed that you have not been home. So stop worrying, when we get there, I will go next door and speak with Mrs. Light and explain the situation."

"Good idea, Rah. That would relieve my mind, you know that I don't trust your father. Also, please don't let me leave there without getting some apples to bring back with us. I have been craving them terribly lately."

"I won't Mom."

"I can't have the Fall season come and not make apple pies no matter what condition I am in."

"Amanda, please watch your brother and sisters for us while we are gone. They are not allowed outside unless you are with them. Kids, mind your sister until we get back. Meme just needs to pick up some clothes and other stuff at her house. Be good."

Chapter 23
My Home

The drive to my home took about ten minutes. Oh how I loved my home. I have lived there for over twenty six years. I raised the children there. They grew into adults in this house. It was our home. It looked very different now, from the way it first looked when we purchased it. But I knew from the moment I walked into the front door and saw the most magnificent fireplace I had ever seen, that house was going to be my home. The house sat on a huge hill in the middle of an apple orchard. It was small, three bedrooms and one bath. But it had all hardwood floors and many windows, which let the sunshine in all day long. I knew from that first look, this is where I belonged. The price was right, we made an offer and the seller accepted it. Within a month, I was in there sanding the floors, painting, and redoing the kitchen cupboards.

As we drive down the long driveway, I see a completely remodeled home. Now, it is a huge barn shaped house with a enclosed sun porch and brand new upstairs living quarters. My heart felt like it was going to jump out of my chest. My heart was broken. The anguish of seeing the house was almost as bad as the cancer. I was going to lose it any day now. That was the reality of it all. My home, my safe place. Going, going gone.

A lump in my throat had already started to choke me. I tried to get my mind off the lump by fumbling for my house keys. Rah reached over and touched me, "Mom, can you handle this?"

I looked at her with the tears already in my eyes and simply said, "I have to. Just give me a minute and I will be fine." We sat there for a minute or two in silence, and then I reached for the door handle and got out of the car. Rah followed me. I unlocked the door and walked in everything looked exactly the same as the morning I had left. I tried to remember what I had been thinking that morning when I had left for work. I do remember feeling very ill, but I had not prepared myself for what was coming by any means. I hadn't stopped and thought about the consequences of my illness. I guess I was just not thinking at all.

I walked straight through the kitchen and passed the dinning room and living room. I did not look left or right. I kept moving down the hall and into my bedroom. My room was painted a pale yellow. The bedspread had brown and yellow designs on it, as did the matching curtains. Very country. My bedroom set was a dark pine, with a hutch type dresser and large hutch mirror sitting on top of the larger dresser. I had two night stands, one of which had a tv and VCR sitting on it. The room was as neat as a pin, if I have to say so myself. I was compulsively neat and my home reflected that.

I walked to my clothes closet and opened the double doors. Once I started going through my clothes, I knew that I was going to have a problem. "Oh Rah, nothing is going to fit me. I've lost so much weight."

"Don't worry, you will gain it back. Just take some of your sweaters and few pairs of pants that you know were too tight for you."

"I will grab you some underwear and some socks." Rah started to go through my bureau drawers searching for the underwear drawer.

"Please take only the really pretty bras and panties Rah. It's all I have left that makes me feel attractive."

"Oh Mom, you still look good. Just a little thin."

"Liar," but thanks."

I placed a pile of sweaters and pants on the bed. There is so much that has to be packed, how was I ever going to manage it all? Twenty six years is a long time to collect things. I thought to myself, *I will only keep what is necessary. Nothing else. Half of my possessions were totally useless and had no monitory value. Just all sentimental junk. But I don't think that I am much different than anyone else. We all keep silly little trinkets that remind us of certain places or people. I believe that a move of this size and all that it entailed would scare the heck out of anyone, either sick or healthy.*

Rah had picked out a few bras and panties and placed them on the bed as well. "Pretty undies, Mother."

"Well don't you get any ideas of borrowing them. Your left breast would fill my entire bra, so forget it."

"Well, I don't want to brag....but."

"Never mind, I don't want to hear it. It was the vitamins I took when I was carrying you, that gave you your figure, so you can thank me for your big boobs." We both started to giggle.

I was very relieved that Rah had come with me, and I had not attempted this myself. I really don't think my state of mind could have handled it. But with Rah here with me, she'll help me get through it even with a laugh. We threw everything into two large black garbage bags. Neither one of us had thought to bring a suitcase. Nevertheless, the garbage bags did what they were supposed to. We carried the two bags to the car. I returned to the patio door to lock the door. "You go ahead and talk to the neighbor and tell her what is going on Rah. I will meet you in the car." For a second I wanted to return inside the house and just sit down at the kitchen table one more time. But the little voice inside me said, better not Pam, just leave now. So I listened to the voice and returned to the car containing the garbage bags and my questionable future and simply leaving my old life behind. I sat there waiting for Rah to finish talking to the neighbor. My neighbor smiled and waved at me. I simply smiled and waved back.

"Want to stop and get something to eat? Are you hungry Mom?

"Actually I am."

"Do you want some soup or something along that line?"

"Goodness no, I have had enough of soup for a while. If I am going to feel this sick to my stomach all the time, I think I deserve to put something in it that I enjoy once and a while. What's the difference? No matter what I eat, it doesn't stay there. Let's stop for pizza at Tony's. That way we can bring a pizza home to the kids. You know that Amanda is not going to cook anything for them."

Tony's Pizza was a short drive from my house. It was like the gathering place for the local town's people. I was a little nervous about going inside because I didn't want to see anyone I knew, but the thought of sitting in the car was the last thing I wanted to do on this beautiful fall day. We went inside, but as luck would have it, no one I knew personally was in there eating . I had to visit the bathroom a couple of times, but for me the pizza was worth it. Rah and I enjoyed our time of being together, and we took the extra pizza we had ordered home with us for the kids.

We pulled into Rah's driveway and was greeted almost instantly by Haley. She spotted the pizza box immediately. "Pizza!"

"Yes little one, we brought one home for you guys."

Tawnee, Amanda and Kyle (name) stayed in the house. They were still playing the game. Amanda was the next one to see the pizza.

"Oh boy, pizza," Amanda said. I am starving."

"Me too," replied Tawnee.

"Not me, I only like hot dogs. I don't like pizza," Kyle name replied.

"Well, I will cook you one in a minute," Rah told him.

"You never have to eat what we eat, you spoiled brat," Tawnee said, totally disgusted."

"Just never mind about him and enjoy the food."

"Meme was nice enough to buy it for you."

"Thanks Meme," echoed from all of them as they happily reached for a piece of pizza.

The kids gathered around the kitchen table, while Rah and I went into the living room. "Mom, why don't you leave some of your clothes up here for now? You know there is no room at Nana's house for them."

"I think your right Rah, I will have some clothes here and some down there. That should work until I move to Brandon's house."

"You have decided to do it then, move to Brandon's?"

"Yes, I think it will be the best for everyone."

"Do you want to phone him and tell him right now?"

"Yea, would you get me the phone, I am feeling a little weak right now. My legs are wobbly. I think I should take a pill."

"Let me get you your pill first, then the phone."

"Oh Rah, we forgot the apples." She looked at me and we both started laughing once again.

I took the pill and then dialed Brandon's phone number. "Thank you for calling...."

"Never mind all that phone technique. This is your mother. How about I come live with you and your family real soon?"

"Are you serious mom?"

" Yes, I have made up my mind."

"That's great mom. I'll call Sue and the kids and tell them right away."

"Brandon, I have a very good idea that I want to discuss with you. I think that it will help you and me at the same time. Why don't you call me tonight when you get home. I will be at Rah's house tonight. I think I might sleep here tonight, if she doesn't mind."

"That's great Mom, I'll call you later."

"Bye son."

"Bye Mom."

Tawnee came running over to me and asked, "Are you going to sleep here tonight?"

"I think I might, if it is okay with your mom and dad?"

"You can sleep with me. Haley can sleep on the couch. Won't you Haley?"

"No dear, I will sleep on the couch, but thank you. Meme is up and down a lot and watches tv until real late."

"Mom, don't be ridiculous, of course you can stay overnight. We would all love to have you here."

"Maybe I can play some more Nintendo?" "What do you think kids?"

Chapter 24

Newspaper Ad

We played Nintendo until I was totally video gamed out. I swear those kids could play all night long. Their patience when it comes to games is totally amazing. If only they had that much concentration when it comes to school work. I will say that both Tawnee and Haley do very well in school. Kyle (name) is still to young, but next year, we will find out fast what his capabilities are. I don't know what a teacher will do to keep him from jumping around. That will definitely be a challenge for any teacher that should have little Kyle (name) for their student.

Conversation was at a minimum between Greg and Rah. I got the feeling that something was going on between them, but I wasn't going to get into it with either one of them. Better left alone, I thought. I tried to ignore the fact that something wasn't quite right, and I settled down on the couch to rest. I am happy to say that their couch is a heck of a lot more comfortable than my mothers.

We watched tv for a while together, and then both Rah and Greg went to bed. I think it was around two o'clock before I finally went to sleep. There were a couple of the old Dracula movies on, which I really enjoyed. October is a great month for horror movies. The different tv stations play them all month long in recognition of Halloween.

The next morning I found out that no one gets up early at Rah's house. They are all late sleepers. A far cry from my Mom and Dads house. When the sun comes up, Dad gets up. It was a nice change though, I just lay there thinking about everything. Last night I had to get up around four o'clock and take some medicine for pain and diarrhea. After I take it, I just remain perfectly still and the pain subsides and the diarrhea using lessens in about an hour. *My mind is never quiet. It is always thinking about all the different situations that were ahead of me that had to be faced. One at a time, Pam. One at a time.*

I was looking forward to talking to Brandon. He hadn't called last night, or if he had tried the line was most likely busy. Tawnee is always on the phone talking to her girlfriends. Even Rah and Greg are great phone conversationalists. Greg is in some type of Fantasy Football league and Rah has a ton of friends she is always talking to.

The phone did not surprise me when it rang at 9:30 a.m., and I knew that it had to be Brandon. " Hello?" I said.

"Mother, I tried to call you last night, but the line was busy all evening."

I tried to keep my voice low as not to wake anyone. "Well, good morning to you to son."

He laughed. "Seriously Mom, I tried all evening."

"I know, but there are a lot of people in this house and unfortunately for us, they all like to talk on the phone. I am not about to tell them to get off, when it's their phone."

"What did you want to discuss, Mom?"

"Okay, here it goes. Bran you know that I have to sell almost everything in the house very soon."

"Yes, I know that."

"What do you think of this? I will put an ad in the paper and have a moving sale. I will keep only the furniture needed for my apartment in your downstairs and sell everything else. The money from everything I sell will be used to pay for all the construction downstairs. Plus with any luck, we will be able to buy carpet, kitchen cabinets, bathroom fixtures. What do you think?"

"Mom, the last thing I want to do is take your money."

"Brandon, listen to me. You will be using the money to make me a home. Why shouldn't I help to pay for it? You think about it, and discuss it with Susan. I truly believe that it is the best for everyone."

"Today I am going to Jays house for dinner, but I will be back to Nanas' house by seven. You can call me then and let me know how you both feel about it.

"Alright Mom. I'll call you after seven tonight. Make sure you don't overdue at Jays' house. Tell Jay and Ann that I said hello, and that they could come and visit once me in a while.

"Okay, Bran, Bye for now, and I will talk to you later on."

"Bye, Mom"

Tawnee was the first one to get up. "I heard the phone ring, was it my friend Angie? Angie was Tawnee's best, best friend.

"No Tawnee, it wasn't her. I am sorry the phone woke you up."

"Oh, I wasn't sleeping, I just didn't want to get up."

Kyle was exiting his room by this time. "Hi Meme."

"Good morning little Kyle(name)."

Next in the room was Amanda. She just walked (perhaps I should say ran) into the bathroom. "Poor kid," I thought. I could hear her gaging. I can tell she didn't take my advice regarding the crackers.

Tawnee said, "Just the sound is making me sick."

Amanda came out of the bathroom and sat down on the love seat. "Amanda, go get a cracker right now. It will help you."

Her hair was all wet from sweating and her face was almost pure white. All you could see was her big blue eyes. She was holding a cold face cloth on her forehead. Put the cloth of the back of your head, on your neck. That will help too."

"I'm so sick, Meme," Amanda said weakly.

"I know, but it will pass. Tawnee, get your sister a cracker from the cupboard." Tawnee moved really quickly and grabbed a box of crackers. "Amanda, just take small bites out of one and then put your head between your legs. It will help you stop the nausea."

"Boy, I am never going to get pregnant, said Tawnee. "I hate throwing up."

Rah made her appearance next. "Feeling sick this morning, Amanda,?" Ra asked.

"Oh yes, Mom." Amanda answered without lifting her head up.

"Make sure you don't put any milk in your stomach. Stick to plain water. If it comes up, it's not so bad." Rah looked over at me and just shook her head.

"Mom, do you want some coffee?"

"Oh yes, definitely. Sorry that I didn't make any, but first Brandon called, and then little miss Amanda needed some assistance."

"Don't worry about that, I thought that I heard the phone. What did Brandon have to say?"

"He is going to talk to Sue and call me tonight. He sounded quite pleased about my proposal."

I had my coffee and Rah also made some toast for me. I had to get myself moving and get back to my mom's house and clean up before Jay came to pick

107

me up. I knew that Jay would be right on time, as was always his way. Prompt and punctual, he hated waiting.

Dad arrived around eleven o'clock. I had thrown on and old bathrobe of Rah's and was out the door quickly after saying my goodbyes to everyone. "Make sure you call me this evening Rah."

"You have a nice time up to Jay's and tell everyone that I said hello."

"I will," and I walked out the door heading for my dad's car.

Dad asked, "did you enjoy yourself?"

"Oh yes, and I slept pretty good. Anytime I can sleep is a good time for me." He smiled at me and proceeded to start the car. Good thing there was nothing seriously wrong with this old piece of junk. It may be old, but it usually gets me where ever I want to go.

We headed for home and while he was driving, he asked, "Did you eat this morning?"

"Only some toast. But that was really all that I could handle this morning."

"What time is Jason coming to pick you up?"

"About noontime."

"I should have plenty of time to get ready before he arrives."

Mom was busy cooking when we walked in the door. Ever since I could remember, we always had a large Sunday dinner. It was a tradition that was never ignored no matter what was going on. "Did you get any rest over there?"was her first question.

"Yes, I did." " The couch was very comfortable."

"You mean one of those kids didn't give you their bed?"

"Oh Mom, of course they offered, but I said no. I have to get up and down so much, no one would have gotten any sleep."

"What time is Jay coming?"

"About noon," I said while I was headed for the bathroom. I needed to get out of my moms way quickly. She was headed for a question and answer period, and that was the last thing I needed this morning. I closed the bathroom door and breathed a sigh of relief.

Emotionally I needed my shower this morning. I grabbed on to the metal bars on the wall and began my routine. The tears helped me emotionally, but they also drained and exhausted me. I had to make sure that I was going to be stable this afternoon visiting Jay. I could not afford to lose control in front of him. I had to be at my best for Jay and wear my happy face. I see no need to give my children any more burdens than they already have. If I showed confidence and strength, so would they. So come on Pam and smile.

After the shower, and making myself look presentable, I returned to the kitchen. I sat down with a piece of paper and began to compose my ad for the furniture sale.

"What are you writing?"my mom asked.

"My moving ad. The ad to sell all my furniture, mom. It has to be done, and I can't put it off any longer.

"I wish that something could be done that you would not have to do this, Pam. It's all you have in the world."

"No kidding Mom. But I have come to the conclusion that they are only material things. Material things can be replaced. When I am well again and on my feet, then I will replace what I need to. Not to worry, Mom. God taught me a very valuable lesson. Your family is the most important thing in your life, not what you own. So everything will work out. I believe that with all my heart. I have to believe that or I couldn't go on. God has his plan for me, and I can only follow it without question."

I finished the ad and read it over. It sounded good. Now if the people just come and buy, I will be in business. I made sure the ad started this coming Friday and ran through the weekend. It was apple time in Clayson, and the town was busy with city people riding through the town, looking at the fall foliage and buying apples. A good time for a moving sale, I thought to myself. I will make sure I have a sign out in front so anyone driving by can see it plainly.

I knew, well almost knew, what furniture I was going to keep. I'll keep the white wicker bedroom set, the double door refrigerator, the tv and maybe the coffee tables. That should fill up a small apartment. I wanted to buy a small living room set, the one that is in my home is much to big to fit downstairs in Brandon's house. Brandon and Sue already had a washing machine and a dryer so therefore mine could be sold. Yes, I think I am getting a handle on this. Now, if I can set some prices in my mind for these pieces of furniture, I will have it made. One less thing to worry about. If I am really lucky, I will have enough money to buy some carpet and bathroom fixtures along with the construction materials.

The doorbell rang, it was Jay. He was right on schedule. I stood up and announced to all, "I am all set to go. "What's for dinner?

Jay replied proudly, "Ann made your favorite, spaghetti and sausage."

"Great, let's get going before little Cheyenne eats it all. Even serious Jay had to crack a smile from that remark. Jay helped me with my coat.

"Bye Mom, see you later on."

Her expected reply was, "Have a nice time, but don't you eat to much or you will be sick."

I turned to Jay as we walked out the door and said, "Like I'm not already sick? We started to laugh when my mother came out the door yelling, "Did you take your pills?"

"Yes Mom, I have them in my pocketbook." I looked at Jay and said, "See, I am 54, and my mom is still looking after me. See what you are in for." We kept on laughing as we approached the car.

It was quite a ride to Jays home and I was a little nervous that I would need to make a bathroom stop, but the medicine did what it was supposed to do. Thank goodness. Jay and Ann lived in a small town right over the Rhode Island state line. The house was very small, but fit their needs. Ann was standing at the window when we pulled in the driveway. She had the baby in her arms.

"Every time I see Ann, she is holding little Cheyenne. Does she ever put her down?"

"Nope, she never does. Cheyenne is pretty spoiled, but what can you do? Ann is a great mother."

We went inside and talked about things in general. I made sure that we stayed away from any talk regarding my illness. Ann out did herself with the meal. She was such a pleasant young girl, but I really didn't know Ann that well. I had not had much of a chance to get to know her as they had a whirlwind romance and married very quickly after a few short months of dating.

Ann had really out did herself. The dinner tasted so good to me. I knew that I would pay for eating Italian food later on tonight, but I couldn't resist. Ann had put so much effort into the meal.

"The meal was wonderful, Ann."

She smiled and said, "Wait until you try my apple pie."

"Apple pie, my favorite."

"I know, Jay told me. I hope you like it. Jay says you make fabulous apple pies."

"I am sure that I will love it Ann. Don't worry so much."

She put the baby to bed, after we had desert. She had held her the entire time we were eating, and little Cheyenne did not make a sound. She just looked around and cooed and smiled. Such a happy little baby, and she looked so much like Jay. I silently gave thanks to God for such a beautiful grandchild. In fact, all my grandchildren were beautiful. I really did have a lot to be thankful for. I have to remember that, when I start to pity myself.

We went into the living room and we watched some fishing program (gee, that's a surprise) and talked a little. "Now is a good time to bring up the furniture sale," I thought. Jay, I put the ad in the paper for the furniture. It starts next Friday and runs through the weekend. I am going to need you there for help. Rah and Brandon will be there. I figure people might need help in carrying things, and stuff like that. "Can you be there?"

"I'll be there Mom, but I can't help but wish that it didn't have to happen."

"I know, it will be hard on all of us. But you know son, that it has to happen. The bank is liable to come and tape off the house so I can't even get in, never mind sell anything. So, I can't wait any longer. It's now or never, I need the money." The thought ran through my mind, *now would be a good time to tell him about me moving in with Brandon and Sue,* but I didn't want to chance ruining the wonderful day we have had. So I kept my secret for a short time longer.

"Do you like living up here Jay?"

"I do, but Ann is not to fond of it," he admitted. It's too far from all her family, and with only one car she doesn't get to see them very much unless they visit us."

"Maybe you could find a place in RI? Even in Johnston? There a lot of apartments there."

"No, I hate the city, Jay said quickly. I need to stay in the country. I want Cheyenne to grow up in the country just like I did. Maybe someday we can afford to buy a house in Clayson. But we're okay here for the time being."

"I know that you have been avoiding talking about your illness, Mom. But, please tell me what is going to happen tomorrow with your Chemo treatments?"

"Well, I have to be there early, and they tell me it takes about four to five hours, then I have to go to the radiation doctor for that treatment. Sounds like a fun day, don't you think?"

"Jay got "that look" on his face, and I knew that I had better say something positive fast. " Now Jay, these treatments are going to cure this cancer. So we have to be thankful that they are available to me. We have to stay in a positive frame of mind. I need you to do that for me. Please? I am going to be fine. I am going to live to see Cheyenne get married."

I quickly changed the subject before Jay could say anything else. "Jay, on the way home, could we stop and buy some apples? "Rah and I both forgot to buy them the other day when I was at the house getting some of my clothes."

"Ann's pie made me think of it."

"Sure Mom, I'll stop that's no problem."

"It's getting kind of late, and I really should be home early. Tomorrow is a big day. Would you mind taking me home now, I am feeling kind of tired? It's a long drive and I don't want to forget my apples again.

"I'll get your coat, mom."

"Ann are you coming for the ride?"

"No, the baby is still asleep. You two go, if I wake her up she will be cranky and we won't have a very enjoyable ride."

"Oh are you sure?"

"Yes, you go, I will call you tomorrow in the afternoon to check up on you."

"Again Ann, thank you for the lovely meal. I truly enjoyed it."

Jay got my coat, I kissed Ann good bye, and I left the house with my son by my side. At first we both were quiet, but Jay broke the silence and asked, "Where do you want to get the apples, Mom?"

"How about Palumbo's Orchard.? They usually have a good assortment on hand."

We pulled into the parking lot of the orchard and Jay asked, "Do you want to go inside and pick out the apples?"

"No, I need to sit here Jay."

"You go in and buy about five pounds of Mac's. They make the best pie as far as I am concerned."

"You should know, your pies were always the best. I loved them when I was a kid."

"Ann's apple pie was very good," I said.

"She used the recipe you gave her when we first were married."

"That is so sweet of her." He smiled and got out of the car.

Jay was only gone a few minutes and returned with his arms full of apples. He looked like my little boy used to after sending him out into our orchard for apples. Big smile, my handsome boy. He got into the car and put the apples on the back seat. "Want one Mom?"

"Yes, I do." When we pulled out of the parking lot, both of us were enjoying a fresh crisp apple together, as we had done so many times before in years gone by.

We got to mom's house right on schedule, about 6:30 p.m. "Do you want to come in?"

"No, I'll pass Mom, but I will carrying the apples for you to the door."

"Thanks for the wonderful day, Jay."

"I love you, and drive carefully."

"Don't worry, I will." He smiled and handed me the bag of apples. "Bye mom."

My mother was sitting in the living room watching her favorite western channel when I came in with the apples. "Did you have a nice day?"

"Oh, yes Mom, I really did."

"Everybody has called looking for you."

"I I told them what time you would be home."

"I'll call them tomorrow."

"How are Jay and Ann doing?"

"Their struggling, but their okay. I brought you some apples."

"Good, I have been in the mood for something sweet all day. I'll make some pies."

"Mom, I want to make the pies."

"No, you rest, I'll make them."

"How about if I peel them, and you make them? That way, you won't be mad with me for over doing?"

Dad came in the kitchen and said laughing, "How about I make the pies and you two go sit in the living room?" Even mom had to laugh at that. So we compromised and I peeled the apples, and she made the crust. No matter how you look at it, we both made the apple pies.

Once the pies were in the oven my attention turned to finding something to wear tomorrow morning. "Where is the garbage bag I brought from the house?"

"Oh, it's in the closet in my bedroom."

"Okay, I'm going to see what I can find that will be suitable for tomorrow." It took me a few minutes, but I found a pretty sweater and a pair of black pants. That will work. I'll shower in the morning, I am too tired tonight. Later on that evening Mom, Dad and myself enjoyed a nice piece of hot apple pie. They went to bed at their usual time and I relaxed on the couch watching tv. Sleep came quickly as my day had been a busy one.

Chapter 25
Chemotherapy

I awoke before anyone this morning. Thankfully, my night had been a restful one. I think that I had been so tired from yesterday, that even the pain was too tired to hurt me. I took my medication and headed for "the shower."

I undressed and stepped in. As the hot water started covering my body, I let myself totally relax. I let the tears come, but I was not sobbing. Not today. Maybe, I was finally running out of tears. I held on to the comforting bars and put my head down to start washing my hair. Suddenly from nowhere the room was spinning. Thank goodness for the bars. I had lost my balance and had it not been for me holding on to them, I would have fell backwards. Where did this come from? I sat down on the shower floor and let the water just fall over me. I just sat there and cried letting the hot water rinse the tears away. I tried to focus on the bath tub knobs and make the dizziness disappear. I don't know exactly how long I sat there, maybe a minute or longer. Then as suddenly as the dizziness had started, it stopped and I started to feel better. I carefully pulled myself up to an almost standing position. Now I was really mad. I had planned to make my hair look especially nice today. I knew that it would be a while before I was going to look normal again, so I wanted today's hair style to be special, no matter how bad I felt. I thought, well, my hair is clean, that's something. I will just do the best I can with it, but it is going to take me longer than usual to get ready. Thank heaven I got up earlier than normal. I shouldn't have taken my medication on an empty stomach. That's why I got so dizzy. Stupid me. I put on my clothes, dried and styled my hair and put on my makeup. As I looked in the mirror, all I could think was, you did a good job. I walked into

114

the kitchen and faced my biggest critic, my mom.

"Well don't you look nice."

I smiled. I had accomplished what I had set out to do. "Thank you, I tried."

"I wouldn't be able to tell that you were sick, if I didn't already know. But, I don't know why you torture yourself everyday with makeup and stuff. Why not just...."

"What, I asked, "Give up? "I just don't think so."

"You know I didn't mean it like that, Pam."

"I know mom, I'm sorry. I am just really scared this morning. I just had to give it my best shot today." Who knows, I may be totally bald tomorrow morning. You know what Dr. Johnson said. Oh God, I should have a wig or something for my head. Right now, I just can't afford a wig. I should have remembered to bring my scarfs from the house with me when I packed. Honestly, sometimes if I had a brain, I would be dangerous."

"Pam, do you want me to go with you today?"

"No, it's best that you don't. Today is going to be an all day thing. First Chemo and then radiation. You probably won't see me again until sometime after three this afternoon. You and Dad just go up to Rah's and help Amanda with the kids this morning and get the girls off to school. Amanda is in no condition right now to deal with her sisters. That will keep Rah from worrying about them all day. Dad, if you could return up there around four o'clock, that's when the girls get home from school, and stay until Greg gets home, it will help out a lot. Would you mind?"

"Of course not, tell Rah not to worry," he replied.

I heard the horn toot, and I knew that Rah was waiting for me. I hugged dad first, and then my mom. "Wish me luck. I love you both. Bye, see you this afternoon." I grabbed my coat and headed out the door.

We arrived at the Women's Center at about 7:45 a.m. We walked in and got on the elevator passing the beautiful fountain. The elevator door opened and I was greeted by the receptionist. "Good morning, Ms Ayer. This morning you have to report downstairs to the lab for your first blood test. I apologize for not telling you about the lab when you were her last week. A blood test has to be done each week before you can receive the Chemo treatment. They are checking your blood constantly for the condition of your blood cells."

"Oh, that's no problem, I replied. Is it on the first floor?

"Yes, just turn right when you get off the elevator. The lab is on your right," she replied. Just give them your name and they will handle it from there."

Rah and I turned around and entered into the open elevator. "This is fun, don't you think, Rah?" "Mom, behave yourself. Don't get me laughing."

The elevator stopped once again and the door opened. We turned to the right as was instructed and there was the lab. It only took a couple of minutes, and the blood was drawn and the test was completed. Back into the elevator again. "Mom, do not say one word."

"I won't I said," wearing my biggest smirk.

Once back in the main reception area, all we could do was sit and wait. I was so frightened, and I know that Rah could sense my fear. She reached over hand held my hand. I was relieved to have her here with me, for I don't know how I could have handled this all alone. I knew that in time, that is what I was going to have to do, but for now I was not alone. It was comforting to have her here with me. Just how long Rah could take the pressure of seeing me ill was the big question. But for now, she was here with me. Thank God.

The reception area was filled with women. But there was not a sign of the young girl that had spoken to me on the very first day. I started praying for her health at that moment, but was interrupted by hearing my name called out.

"Ms. Ayer?"

I stood up, "Yes."

"Please come with me."

I looked at Rah and said, "Here I go."

She never let go of my hand. We followed the woman and were escorted into one of the rooms that hand a lounge recliner, tv, VCR and a large bathroom. I sat in the recliner and waited. Rah sat just a few feet away from me in the corner. My heart was pounding and I was sure that Rah could see it beating through my sweater.

A young black woman came in and asked, "May I get you anything right now? A drink of juice, some toast or anything else?"

"No, I am fine." I don't think I could have swallowed anything at that very moment. I gave her a weak smile. I thought it best to admit my fear and simply said, "I am scared to death."

She placed her hand on my shoulder and said, "I know, I really do. You will be fine. Try not to worry to much." She handed me the tv remote and said, "We have a good selection of movies, if you can't find anything interesting on the tv. I will go and get you the list."

I looked at Rah, she looked just as surprised as I felt. "A movie list?"

"I guess so Mom. That's a great idea." Rah said. Sure enough, the young black girl returned with a small booklet full of movie titles. "Can you imagine? Pick one Mom."

I was too nervous to even hold it, as how my hands were shaking. I handed the list to Rah, and said, "You pick."

A second nurse came in the room and simply stated, "Your blood test came back. Are you ready to start the treatment?"

"Yes, I want to get it started."

"First, comes the IV. I am going to put it into your hand. Are you right handed or left handed?"

"Right."

"Okay, then I will put it in your left hand. It will be easier for you if your good hand is not hurting. Once the IV is in place, we can start the drips of your chemo. If you get weak or woozy from a needle, just look away. I'll be quick."

"No, needles don't bother me." I will say she knew what she was doing, one pinch and she was finished.

"And now, the good stuff begins," she said smiling. She had three different bags of medicine on a rolling pole of some sort. I have no idea, what it is called, the pole that its. All three bags had my name on them. She explained that one bag was the chemo itself, one was medicine to keep me from getting nauseous and the last guarantee was a simple saline solution to keep up my strength. "Here we go." She plugged them all into the IV that she had placed in my hand. The machine automatically started clicking. I don't know what I expected, perhaps I thought I would feel the chemo going into my body, but I felt nothing.

Rah picked out the movie "The Matrix." The nurses kept coming in checking on me, and we all commented on how cute Kenu Reeves was. The brown haired nurse, Nancy, kept coming in checking the machine. "Do you have any questions?" she asked.

"Yes, what do you advise me to do regarding my hair? Should I shave it all off tonight, when I get home, or wait until it starts to fall out?"

"Don't shave your head. You don't know for sure that your hair is going to fall out."

"But Dr. Johnson told me that I would lose all my hair. In fact, that was the first thing that he said to me."

She gave me a disgusted look and said, "Honey, the doctors don't know everything. Each patient has a different reaction. Each chemo dose is different for everyone. It depends on a lot of different things. Take the wait and see attitude. If your hair begins to fall out, and you want to shave it, go ahead. But don't do it yet. Give yourself a chance, if after three treatments you still have a full head of hair, I can guarantee you, that it's not going to fall out as a result of the chemo."

"I was shocked." Not that I wanted my hair to fall out, but I had never considered that it wouldn't. And so I sat there with my daughter, watching the poison in the bag drip slowly into my body. I was praying that it was going to kill the cancer inside me.

I could hear voices in the hallway and I knew that the other treatment rooms each had other sick women in them. I am sure that they we praying the same prayer, that the treatments would work for them. Just then a young tall blonde girl came in with some juice and a banana for me. "You should really drink this and try and eat some of the banana." She seemed very caring and pleasant. In fact all the people in here were the same way. It was very comforting for me to be surrounded by such nice people.

"What should I do if I have to go to the bathroom?" I asked.

"Just pull the rolling gadget right along with you, it has wheels. But be careful not to pull the IV out."

"Thank you,"I said. She smiled and left the room.

We watched the entire movie which was about two and a half hours long. But the medicine was still dripping into me. The bags were not empty yet. The girl with brown hair came in and checked the medicine. "Just a short time left and you'll be all through for today." She handed me a paper with a list of instructions (mostly do's and don'ts) to use as a guide when I returned home. I explained to her that I had to report for my radiation treatments as soon as I left here.

"Oh that's no problem. When did you start the radiation treatments?"

"Last week on Friday, officially."

"Usually they wait for the chemo treatments to begin first, but the doctor must want to get a jump on us, she said smiling. Did he explain to you just how the chemo works with the radiation?" "Yes, pretty much. I think I understand it. He said, "The chemo prepares the cells to accept the radiation quicker. Also, that the two work together, and can usually do serious damage to the cancer cells."

"Yes, he explained it well. Now you sit back and talk to your daughter, or call a friend. That is what the phone is for. It is there for your use and your convenience. I'll be back in a short while to see if you are finished. If the machine starts to buzz, don't get nervous. It's just notifying me that you are finished."

"Kind of like a microwave oven? I'm done when it dings?"

She smiled and replied, "I guess you could put it that way. You have a great since of humor."

"You've got a funny mom."

"Tell me about it,"Rah replied.

The minutes seemed to drag by and finally the machine started to buzz. The nurse came in shortly and checked all the bags of medicine. "Yes, little one, your through." She unhooked the IV from my hand. A huge black and blue mark was beginning to show. "See, I told you everything would go fine. Any questions?"

"No, I don't think so."

"Well, if you should think of one after you get home, call the number on the top of the list I gave you, as someone will be here to answer any question that you may have." She patted me on the shoulder and left the room.

"Come on Rah, we have just enough time to get to Fairfield without being late." It was already 1:30 in the afternoon. I had no idea that it would take so long for the chemo treatments. Rah did remind me that Dr. Johnson had told her that it could take four or five hours, but I had totally forgotten his advice and comments. Rah helped me out of the chair and I took my coat and purse. "Come on daughter dear. Let's make our escape right now." Everyone said goodbye as we walked down the hall headed for the double doors and the elevator.

The receptionist just smiled and said, "I have your appointment card for you. We will see you next Monday at the same time." I took the card, smiled, and the elevator doors opened.

Chapter 26
Double Dose Day

Rah and I pulled in the parking lot of the Radiation building right on schedule. I asked Rah, "Are you hungry?"

"Yea, kind of, Mom."

"Why don't you go get yourself something to eat while I am inside getting my treatment? You can bring me back some food, so I can eat when I get done. It's not going to take very long here. At least I don't think so. Nothing like the chemo treatments. No five hours here, that's for sure."

"Are you sure that you don't want me to go in and wait?"

"No, that is silly. I have to do this alone, they won't let you in when I get the radiation. You just go and get yourself some lunch. By the time you are finished eating, I will have had my treatment. I know what to expect in here and unless something unforseen goes on, I will be done in a flash. She finally agreed with me, and I stepped out of the car. See you in a bit."

In the lobby there were no patients waiting. I walked passed the receptionist, said my hello and continued down the hall to the locker room. I opened my locker, took out my personalized dressing gown and slipped it over my head. I neatly hung up my sweater and pants and closed the locker door.

The patient lounge was quite. There was no tv running, and there was only one patient sitting there quietly reading a book. She looked up and smiled, I smiled back as I chose which chair to sit in. I would guess that she was anywhere from thirty to thirty five years old. She spoke first. "Hello, my name is Jane Thomas."

"Hi, I am Pam Ayer."

"It's nice to meet you, Pam. It would be nicer if we could meet under different circumstances, don't you think? she continued.

"Yes, I have to agree with you there."

"Would I be to nosey if I asked you what was wrong, and what you were receiving radiation treatments for?" she asked.

"Oh no," I replied. "Cervical Cancer."

"I have a tumor in my vagina."

"I have Cervical Cancer too. Did you have to have a hysterectomy?"

"No, they decided not to do that, as my cancer has not spread anywhere else. Just the tumor itself is cancerous."

"Oh, she said quietly. My cancer spread to my uterus. So, they took everything out. Now, I can't have any children."

"Oh, I am so sorry." was all that I could say. I couldn't help but notice that she was wearing a wig, and not a very good one. It's a good guess on my side to say that the wig she was wearing was in my price range. That is to say if I had a price range, which of course I did not.

Still curious, she asked, "Have you started your Chemo treatments yet?"

"Yes, I had my first treatment this morning," I replied. "Today is only my second radiation treatment."

"Are you feeling sick yet?"

"No, not yet anyways."

"Are you going to wear a wig, or a hat when your hair falls out?" she asked.

"I haven't decided as yet."

"Well, you should really give it some thought, as the hair goes pretty fast."

"It's quite devastating."

"I have been thinking about it, but I think that I can handle it when it happens, " I answered.

I asked how her how the treatments were going?"

She quickly responded, "Not very well. I just keep hoping that the cancer won't spread anywhere else. I have had so many Chemo and radiation treatments, that I have lost count."

A nurse appeared at the door and announced, "Ms. Thomas, we are ready for you, come along."

She got up off the chair and turned to me and said, "Good luck and maybe we can talk again soon."

"Good luck to you to June," was all I could say.

I sat and waited until the nurse came after me. She smiled and commented,

"My, don't you look nice today."

"Thank you, I try very hard to keep up appearances."

"That is very important you know," she replied. It is not only important for you, but believe it or not it helps the other patients as well. Besides the better we women look, the better we feel, right?" "Right, I said smiling.

"Did you have your Chemo treatment this morning?"

"Yes, I did."

"How are you feeling?"

"Not too bad, at least not right now? How did you know that I had my Chemo."

"I noticed your left hand, it's turning black and blue. That's always a sign of Chemo. Besides, we keep close track of all your treatments. Dr. Merrick is very thorough with monitoring his patients. I'll give you a little advise. Follow his instructions to the letter. He saved my life, I have been where you are standing." I looked at her and she gave me a wink.

As we walked in to radiation treatment room, I saw Dr. Merrick looking at the machine. "Hello Ms. Ayer, how did you do this morning?"

"Fine, I think."

"I knew you would, he responded. Come on up on the table so we can get you out of here and you can go home and rest, as I am sure that you have had a long day." The nurses prepared everything and Dr. Merrick just stood and oversaw the entire procedure. It was very comforting knowing that he cared enough to make sure that things were done according to his expectations. The treatment was over quickly and I slid off the table. "Still feeling okay?," he asked.

"Yes, but am I supposed to be looking for any side effects? What am I supposed to be expecting?"

"Usually diarrhea or some discomfort urinating, and sometimes nausea. If any of these symptoms cause you serious discomfort, please call this office right away."

"Well Dr Merrick, I suffer from diarrhea all the time anyway."

"Are you taking any medicine for it?"

"Only the over counter stuff, but I am afraid to take it too often. I worry that it will hurt me."

"Don't worry about that, those over the counter pills will not hurt you. If they help, you take them whenever you feel the need. That's it for today, you can go and get dressed."

"Alright Dr., Thank you."

I returned to the locker room and changed my clothes. I hung up my little dressing gown and then checked myself in the mirror. *Ugh!*, I thought to myself. *At least I still have my hair, at the moment anyway. I checked all over my sweater for tell tales signs of hair, but there were none there. So far so good.* I took my purse and coat from the locker, and headed out the door. Dr. Merrick was standing at the Patients Lounge talking to a patient when I walked by. "Ms. Ayer, I wanted to tell you how nice you looked today."

"Well, thank you Doctor. I'll see you tomorrow."

He smiled and I continued on my way out to the front reception area.

Rah's car was parked right out in front of the building. I waved at her from inside the reception area and headed for the outside. Suddenly on my way down the cement walkway, I began to feel very faint. I stopped for a second and held on to the railing. I took a couple of deep breaths. I sure hope that Rah remembered to bring me some food. All these different drugs being put into me, without any food, was not doing me any good. I need food! Rah jumped out of her car and came running in my direction. I put my hand up and said, "I'm okay. I just need some food. Give me a minute, I will be fine." We waited standing there for a minute or two, and then started again for the car.

"Can you make it, Mom?"

"Yes, I am better right now." When I got into the car, Rah handed me a bag containing a roast beef sandwich and some french fries. "Oh, I am so hungry Ra. Thank you so much. I immediately bit into the sandwich and shoveled down some french fries. Apparently my eyes are bigger than my stomach as I hadn't eaten that much when I already felt full. "You can start the car, I really want to go home, it's been a long day."

"Are you sure you wouldn't rather eat while we are parked?"

"No, I said, that is silly, let's get going."

We hadn't been on the road for five minutes when I knew that I had made another mistake. "Rah, I think I am going to be sick."

"What?"

"I think I am going to toss my cookies." She pulled the car over in a flash. It's a wonder we didn't get in an accident, she pulled over so fast. I put my head down between my legs and took deep breaths.

"Are you okay, is there anything I can do?"

"Is there anything to drink, I am so thirsty?," I said with my head still down.

"Yes, I got you a coke rather than coffee. I didn't think coffee would be very good for your stomach." She reached over in the back seat and pick up a bottle of coke from the floor. "Here Mom, take a sip." I took a couple of swallows and just continued with my deep breathing. The nausea passed, it seemed like an hour, but I know that it was only a few minutes.

"Let's go now Rah, before I get sick again."

"Do you think you can manage?"

"Yes, let's just get home."

We were in front of my mothers apartment within ten minutes, and I had managed to keep everything in my stomach. Rah parked the car and ran around to my door. "Rah, I am so sorry to put you through this."

"Don't be ridiculous Mom, like you didn't take care of me when I was a kid, and I was sick. My turn to take care of you. Come on Mom, I'll help you inside."

Chapter 27
Busy, Busy, Dizzy

Rah and I made it into the apartment carrying my roast beef sandwich and coke. My father was sitting in the chair reading the newspaper and mom was in the kitchen cooking. "Your home early," Dad said. "I was just getting ready to go up to your house Rah, and wait for the girls to get home from school."

I reached for the arm of the couch which was right to my left and sat down. I was getting the feeling that it was time to put my head down again. My mom had already made her way into the living room and was just about to say something, when she saw me sitting there.

"Oh God ! What's wrong? Is she sick? she asked Rah. "I knew this was going to happen, I just knew it. She's to frail to handle all these treatments. They are going to kill her."

I looked up and calmly said to her, "Mom, I am alright. It's not from the treatments. I was just hungry and ate the food that Rah got me too fast. That's all it is. Calm down."

My mom insisted, "It's more than that, and your not telling me. Your trying to hide the truth from me. I know it."

"Your wrong, Mom," I said. I just ate too fast. The treatments haven't seem to bother me at all, at least not yet anyway."

Mom was getting herself all worked up. "Look at your hand. Who did that to you?"

Dad spoke up, "Calm down and let her relax a minute will you, for God's sake."

"Nana, it was the food. She got sick right after eating it. Then, Rah repeated Dad's request, " Just calm down."

I lifted my head and relaxed back on the couch. "I'm feeling better now, Mom."

"Well, what did you eat that made you sick?"

Rah spoke up, "I bought her a roast beef sandwich."

"That wasn't very smart of you. You should have bought her some soup. A roast beef sandwich? Don't you ever use your brain?"

"Guess it is time for me to go home now," Rah said picking up her purse.

"Yes Rah, that is a good idea."

"Tawnee and Haley will be getting home from school any minute now." I smiled and winked at her and I know that she got my meaning.

"I'll call you later on Mom."

"Okay and thanks for today Rah."

"Your welcome."

"Bye Gramps, bye Nana." She turned and made a fast exit.

"Mom, you shouldn't have jumped all over Rah like that. It wasn't her fault."

My mother was nervous now, "I didn't mean anything by it, I was just scared when I saw you sitting on the couch in the that condition."

"I know that Mom, but you should call Rah later on and apologize. "She was wonderful to me today." I thank God that she was with me."

"I am sorry, Pam."

My mom had tears in her eyes. "I'll call her a little later on, but for now, can I get you anything?"

"No, I just need to sit her a while. I am starting to feel better now."

"I want you to tell me all about the chemotherapy, as soon as your up to it?"

"I will mom. "Don't worry, I will explain it all to you."

Dad interrupted, "Why don't you leave her alone and just let her rest?"

"Oh for goodness sake, she is my daughter. I'm worried about her."

I looked at Dad and shrugged my shoulders, and gave him a weak smile.

"I'm okay Dad, please don't argue over me."

I remained on the couch for about a half an hour, until I thought things seemed to be settled down. I walked into the kitchen where my mom was setting at the table. "Are you feeling better now, Pam?"

"Yes mom, much better."

"Do you have any soup? I asked. That brought about a big smile from my mother, and she was up and looking in the kitchen cupboards before I finished asking the question. "I knew that you should have had soup." she said firmly. I watched her hustle about the kitchen preparing my soup and thought to myself, "She just worries so much about me. It is not her fault that she doesn't know how to show it." Before I knew it, I had a hot bowl of soup with crackers and a cup of tea sitting in front of me staring up at me from the table.

The clock said 6:15 p.m. when the phone rang. I was just starting to doze off again. Startled, I jumped and ran for the phone. Dizziness came over me once again, and I grabbed for my mom's

rocking chair and sat down with the phone receiver in my hand. "Hello," my voice shaking.

Mom, is that you?" It's Brandon.

"Yes, it's me, I was just taking a little nap."

"How did it go today? Are you feeling okay?"

" It went very well, Bran, considering everything. But, it just takes so long for the chemotherapy treatments. It takes hours, but Rah and I watched the movie *"The Matrix"* during the treatment. That helped the time pass."

"A movie, that's pretty cool Mom."

"Yes, they treat every patient extremely well. I can have food, or even a massage, if that's what I want."

"It sounds like a fancy hotel to me."

"Not quite Brandon, but they are very thoughtful regarding the patients feelings. Right now, I am sitting waiting for my hair to start falling out, some hotel." There was a bit of silence on the other end of the phone caused some concern. "Brandon, that is supposed to be funny."

"I am not laughing Mom. Sue went out pricing wigs for you today. She found a salon that donates wigs to cancer patients. What do you think about that?"

"Well, tell Sue I thank her very much for her thoughtfulness. But, the nurse told me today, that I might not lose my hair. Right now I want to wait and see if I am lucky enough not to lose it. The nurse advised me to wait until I have at least three chemo treatments, and if my hair doesn't fall out, then the chances are excellent that it's not going to. So keep your fingers crossed for me."

"Oh we all will mom, we all will."

"Sue and I decided that this weekend she is going to ask her brother to borrow his truck. That way we can move your bedroom furniture over here on Saturday. You can start staying here this weekend."

"Oh Brandon, what can I say?"

Don't say anything Mom. We'll handle everything. "You go and get some rest, and I will call you tomorrow."

"Yes, tomorrow will be a better day, I only have radiation treatments tomorrow and for the rest of the week." I knew that Brandon would handle things for me. He is such a good son. I can rest easier now. I was thinking about everything just before he called me. *I couldn't even imagine how I was going to handle all of this. Today was only the first day of double treatments. I know I am looking at months and months of treatments. How do people handle situations like this when they are all alone? God has got to be there to help them along. No one could handle this totally alone.*

Ten minutes passed and the phone rang again. This time it was my son Jay. Mom got to the
phone before I could. I motioned for her to give it to me, and she put her hand over the receiver saying, "your tired."

"Not too tired to talk to my children."

"Hi Jay."

"Hi mom, are you doing alright?"

"I'm doing good right now, just resting."

"Have you got everything you need?"

"Yes, I am all set."

"Stop worrying."

"I was concerned that you might be sick. My friends aunt had chemo treatments for cancer and she was very sick all the time."

"The nurses told me today, it all depends on the type of chemo a patient receives. Some get much more ill than others."

"For me, so far so good."

"Great," he replied. Mom, what time do you want me at the house on Saturday?"

"Better be there early Jay, around 9:00 a.m. "I put the sale time starting at 10 a.m. in the paper, but you know how people are. Some will come early thinking that they will be able to buy all the good stuff before anyone else gets there."

"Okay mom, I'll be talking to you again tomorrow. I just wanted to tell my boss about Saturday. You get a good nights rest tonight Mom."

"I'll will, love you."

"Bye mom."

The next call came at eight o'clock. It was Rah. "Hi mom. How's it going? Any hair on the pillow yet?"

"Nope, not one strand. "Things are looking up, Rah. Either that or I am going to wake up balder than an eagle."

"Mom, be serious."

"Alright, alright. Brandon called earlier and Sue found a place that donates wigs to people who have cancer. So I have a back-up, just in case it does all fall out."

"Did he tell what the name of the place was?"

"No, I didn't ask. I just hope that it looks better than the one I saw on a patient today."

"What do you mean?" Rah asked.

"We really didn't have much of a chance to talk this afternoon. But I will explain when I see you tomorrow morning."

"I'll be there early. Try and get some rest mom."

"I will." Bye for now and I love you."

"Bye mom."

My mother came in the living room to check on me before she went to bed. "Mom, can you sit down over here for a minute?"

She gave me a curious look but came over to me and sat down on the couch. "What is it?"

"It's just that I never tell you how much I love you Mom."

"Oh Pam don't, not now."

"I have too." Poor mom, she was already crying. That is not what I had wanted to happen. "Mom, I really need to say this while I have the courage. You have been a wonderful mother, and I love you. I just wanted you to hear that from me. Always remember that. You have always been there for me, no matter what. You and Grama taught me what a mother's love is. That is why I am the person that is sitting next to you today. "Thank you. Now you go to bed, and get some rest. I am fine. I have placed all my faith in God, and he will see us through this. My life is not over yet, and I believe that God has a plan for me, I just don't know what it is as yet. I want you to promise me, that you will be strong and believe that I am in God's hands."

"I love you too, Pam," my Mom said crying.

"I know, I have always known that. Go and get some rest and let us be thankful for these treatments, as I know they are going to help me." She hugged me, and walked into her bedroom. I positioned myself on the couch, and said a prayer. My eyes closed and off to dreamland, I went.

Chapter 28
Time to Panic

I took my pain medication right on time this morning, but I really needed a nerve pill more than the pain medication. I knew that today was going to be the day to discuss leaving Moms' nest and moving to Brandon's house. *Thank heavens for my pills*, I thought. They are called " *Xanax.* " For years I suffered from what was eventually diagnosed as panic attacks. It is a strange thing about panic attacks; they never occur someone would expect. I can never recall coming close to having a panic attack when any sort of crisis was happening in my life. Being a mother of three children, I know about all sorts of crisis. Broken arms, high fevers, broken hearts, etc. These panic attacks would strike me at the least logical time. Sometimes I would wake from a sound sleep with one. Other times, I would be watching tv and an attack would come over me. I never knew when or where the panic would strike.

I used to believe I was dying. I couldn't breath, or swallow, and my heart would be racing so fast that I was sure I was having a heart attack. The first attack I can recall was at the age of eighteen. I had just got married. (That should have been my first clue as to why I was susceptible to the panic attacks.) But in all honesty, it has been suggested by the medical profession that panic attacks are genetic. Anyway, there were countless trips to emergency rooms, sometimes even in the middle of the night. The doctors would always send me home after numerous tests with the diagnosis that there was nothing wrong with me. I thought that I had to be crazy if there was nothing physically wrong with me. Even my family physician, Dr. Trott, would just pat me on my shoulder and write out a prescription of "Valium." He would simply say, "Pam, just go home and rest."

As the years pasted, I came to learn how to live with these attacks. It is called avoidance. If I had an attack in the supermarket, simple, don't go back. If I had one on the highway, I would only drive on the side roads. It finally reached the point, when my children were young, I found myself totally housebound. Of course the kids didn't know that I had a problem; they just accepted me for the way I was, and thought all mothers must be like that. But one afternoon as I was watching tv, I saw a panel of people on a random talk show talking about the very same symptoms that I had. I will never forget that day. After the show was over, I called Dr. Trott with the name of the medicine that these people had been taking. The rest is history. He put me on the drug (Xanax) and I slowly started living again and enjoying life. My confidence level improved and I could enjoy my children and go places with them without fear. Once I was put on the medication, the feeling that I was about to have an attack, left me. I still occasionally think that I might be close to approaching an attack, but the Xanax seems to be able to stop the attack from occurring. It has been a life saver for me, and allowed me to function normally without anyone even suspecting that I ever had such a horrible malady. So this morning, I shall take a Xanax (I am down to taking only one pill every now and then), and I am going to need one for this upcoming talk with my Mom. To complicate matters even more, my dream last night was a terrifying nightmare. I can only remember bits and pieces of it, but my ex-husband was standing in front of me wearing his correctional officers uniform with the cruelest look on his face. A light was hanging over my head and I was seated in a wooden chair. I can remember saying over and over, "I don't know, I don't know." He was relentless, repeating his questions over and over, screaming at me. I was crying hysterically, begging him to stop. That is what must of awakened me. My eyes were filled with tears, and my entire body was soaked from sweat. Not a good dream. But for now, that is all I can remember about the dream, and hopefully as the day wears on the entire dream will leave my thoughts just as he has left my life. I won't think about it now, I think about it...

I turned my thoughts of the dream to another situation entirely. I thought of my hair. Should I look on the pillow and see how much is lying there? Do I dare touch my head? I slowly let my eyes move to the pillow. There was nothing there. I raised my arm and concentrated hard to force my hand to touch my head. "Yes!" I said out loud. My hair was still there. I have made it through the first treatment with no hair loss. Miracles do happen.

Chapter 29

Mother Daughter Talk

Upon my early morning wakening, I discovered that my Mom and Dad had not gotten out of bed this morning as yet, and the available time was used to get into the bathroom first. I undressed and stepped into the shower. The hot water felt wonderful. I really wanted to wash my hair this morning, but I was very leery to cover my head with shampoo. I thought, what if I start scrubbing my head and my hair starts sticking to my hands? If I wash it, is that when the hair comes out, not when your sleeping? I will never know, if I don't try I can't go around with dirty hair, so I took the shampoo bottle and gave it a good squeeze, letting the shampoo drip into my hair. I began to gently rub the shampoo in and then slowly pulled my hands down to eye level. Once again, there was no hair on my hands. I turned my eyes to the floor of the shower, scanning the drain and entire stall, and once again, no hair. "Thank you God for this gift!" There will be no tears this morning. I just have to clean out my thoughts and erase the nightmare regarding my ex. I shall just block it out, and face today with thankfulness. After all, he can't hurt me anymore, at least not like he used too.

I got dressed and continued with my new daily routine. As I opened the bathroom door, I knew that I could smell fresh coffee perking. Good old Dad. Bless his soul. I sat down at the table and the first thing he said was, "Sorry about your mother yesterday Pam."

"It's alright Dad, she means no harm. I know that is just the way she is." While I was waiting for him to pour me a cup of coffee, I thought to myself this would be a good time to tell him about my move to Brandon's house. "Dad, I have decided to stay at Brandon's house. He has already made me a bedroom in his downstairs. He has been working his tail off, these last few days. He showed me the finished room the other day, after my radiation treatment. When he is finished with all the work, I will have a complete apartment with a bedroom, bath, kitchen and living room. I want your opinion. "What do you think?"

Dad answered my question quickly, "I think, if that is what you want, you should do it. Just one question Pam."

"Yes, go ahead" I said.

"Where is he going to get the money for all this construction?"

"I have decided to give him some of my money that I get from the sale of my furniture."

"Dad, I can stay at Brandon's house, it is so close to my radiation treatments. It will save everyone a lot of bother. It will give Rah a break, plus you won't have to go to her house every morning to watch the kids. I think it would be best for me to stay either here or at Rah's house on the weekends for my Monday Chemo treatments. Doing it like that, Rah will only have to bring me one day."

"It sounds like you have it all figured out," he stated.

"I truly think it's the best for everyone,"I replied. Mom won't get herself all worked up worrying about me. I am so afraid that she will have another heart attack. What she doesn't see, won't hurt her, and Dad you know that I am going to get a lot worse before I get better."

He frowned and said, "You know that she is not going to like it."

"I know Dad, I know, but I truly believe that I am doing the right thing."

He smiled and said, "I think you are too. Good luck telling your mother."

"Thanks Dad, I am going to need it. I knew that you would understand. Just stay on my side no matter what she says, or how much she cries."

"I will, don't worry," and he began to cook breakfast.

Mom joined us in the kitchen. She was wearing her usual old worn old pajama's. I buy her new pajamas every birthday and Christmas, but she always goes back to these horrible, ragged

looking pj's, plus she had a white hair net over her head. I smiled at her and said, "You look marvelous, simply marvelous Mom." I know that she didn't get it, which made me laugh even harder.

"Will you stop laughing at me, honestly you and your brother are just alike."

"I am not really laughing at you. Just your outfit."

"Well, if your brother were here, he would be laughing even harder than you."

"I don't how you can be so happy, it's beyond me," she said shaking her head.

"Oh Mom, come over and sit down and join me and Dad for coffee."

"Hmm," was her answer. "You had better eat something this morning besides toast." I don't want to worry about you not eating."

"Okay Mom, I will."

"Plus you will be happy to hear that I have already taken my medication."

"Stop worrying." I remained quiet for a while and let my mother chatter on about the bingo this afternoon in the residents hall across the street.

"You know, your father is going to call the bingo today," she said proudly.

"Well you should definitely win, Mom."

"We would never cheat." she said disgusted.

"I'm teasing you again, Mother."

"Dad, you better be careful or the old ladies will throw their bingo markers at you if you call the numbers too fast." Dad just laughed and continued doing the dishes.

It's now or never Pam. Talk to her now. Just go for it. "Mom, I have been wanting to talk to you about something important."

She looked at me, with a frightened look. "It's not something about the cancer is it? No Mom, it's something I have been talking with Brandon about.

"Just what does Brandon want?"

"Mom, he wants me to come and live with him."

"He what?" was her quick reaction.

"Now before you get all excited, hear me out. I know how you feel about Susan, but Brandon has already finished a bedroom for me in his downstairs. I's beautiful. He took me downstairs to see it as a surprise the first day of my radiation treatment." My Mom just sat there listening to me being very quiet. "He is planning to make an entire apartment downstairs for me. When he is finished, I will have a bedroom, bath, kitchen and living room. Plus, I will have my own entrance."

"Tell me Pam, just where is he getting the money to do all this?"

"I am going to invest the money from the sale of my furniture to help pay for all the construction materials. If I don't have enough, the first thing that he will do is put in a bathroom because of my stomach problem. I can live with that. He'll finish it bit by bit if that is what it takes. So Mom, what do you think? Before you say anything, remember that my radiation doctor is right down the road from Brandon's house, and I will have to go every day for the next five or six months. My staying there will take a lot of pressure off Dad and Rah, and you."

She just sat there for a minute and then finally spoke, "I know that your right about staying there for now Pam, but investing your money in his house is something totally different."

"Mom, I have to live somewhere. I have no money coming in, so I can't rent an apartment. I can't live with Rah, she has too many people there now. In addition, Amanda is having a baby. Where the heck would she put me? I can't stay here, you and Dad would get yourself in trouble with the Housing Authority. Whose left, Jay? He lives in Connecticut, how would I get to the doctors? Plus Jay has only one car." My Mom didn't say a word, she just kept looking at me. "You know I am right, and I am making sense. Brandon"s offer is the best way for me to go. It's the best for everyone involved, especially me. Sue will be there to help me, if I get sick. So Mom, what do you think?"

"I think that you have already made up your mind, that is what I think."

"I will still be staying here or up to Rah's on the weekends. That way Rah can bring me to my Chemo treatments every Monday and Sue can bring me every day to the radiation treatments."

"I talked about it this morning with Dad, he agrees with me."

"So…?"

Mom finally spoke, "I think if it is what will make things easier for you, do it. I know that it has to be difficult for you to live out of a garbage bag like you have been doing. I just worry about you. Suppose things don't work out at Brandon's house? You know what type of people Susan's family are. " "There is something strange about them."

"But Mom, I will be in my own apartment downstairs. They won't bother me."

My Mom sighed and said, "Okay, you do what you have to do. I'll go along with whatever you decide."

"Thanks Mom, I really need you to understand. I don't think I could handle having you upset with me right now."

"Tell me, when will this move take place?" she asked.

"This weekend, I think? I know for sure that my bedroom will be moved into Brandon's house on Saturday. I'll probably take all my clothes as well. Then it's settled Mom? Your okay with it?"

"Yes, Pam, I am fine with it."

I finally changed the subject. "Mom you didn't notice but my hair is still here.

None of it fell out last night. The nurse at the Women's Center told me that it might not, and so far she was right. Brandon told me that Susan found a place that would supply me with a wig for free, if I need one."

"That was very thoughtful of Susan," my mom admitted. "

"Yes, it was. Well, I better get moving, Rah will be here shortly. I walked over and gave my Mom a hug. "Want some more coffee, Mom?"

"No thanks," was all she said.

Rah was right on time. She rang the bell and then walked in. Dad was already dressed and ready to go up to her house and get the girls ready for school. Things seem to be proceeding like clockwork. *"Thank you God*, I thought.

"Are you ready to go Mom?" Rah asked.

"Yes, I am all set. Is Amanda up so that she can give Dad some help?"

"I made sure of it. Not to worry," Rah smiled. I took my coat and we were off and running one more time.

Chapter 30
Another Day, Another Pain Pill

Rah and I both were very quiet on route to the doctors office. I knew that Rah was very tired, although she would never admit it to me. I had put an excessive amount of pressure on her over the last few weeks, and I kept thinking, *it will get easier soon Rah. Just hang in there a little while longer for me.*

Rah suddenly broke the silence and said, "Mom, I have to pay my cable bill today while you are at the doctors. They have a payment center in the Mall, and if I don't pay the bill today the kids will

never forgive me. They have to have their cable or their lives would be devastated."

"I know exactly how they feel," I said smiling. You just do what you have to do, and if I am not finished when you get back here, don't sit in the car and wait. Go over to Susan's and wait. I'll call you. It's much too cold to sit in a car and wait." She agreed and promised to do as I suggested.

"How is the money situation at your house?" I inquired.

"About the same as always, we rob Peter to pay Paul. That system seems to keep us afloat every month."

I smiled, "that is what old Grama used to say. It seemed to work for her."

"Well, Greg and I are young, so we are confident things will improve over time. Besides Mom, I am tough just like you taught me to be. I don't want you worrying about me Mom. You have enough on your mind right now."

"Alright, I won't worry at all about you, how's that?" I asked smugly.

"Very funny, Mom."

But before the conversation was finished I had one more question. "How are things between you and Greg,? I noticed some tension in the air the other night when I slept over. Oh, he was just in one of his moods. It had nothing to do with you being there if that is what you are thinking. He really loves you Mom. So just get that out of your mind right now!."

I smiled, and some of my concern regarding their relationship relaxed, at least for the time being.

"How's your pain today, Mom?"

"About the same," I answered. Sometimes it hurts so much, I think that dying would be a relief," I confessed.

"Mom, don't say things like that. I can't stand it when you talk like that."

"I am sorry Rah, but sometimes I can relate to why people commit suicide. I am sure that sometimes it is not for themselves, but a release for their family members."

"Mom, if you continue to talk like that, I will kill you myself."

We both started laughing at that statement, and all I could say in between the laughter was, "Gee thanks Rah, you are so thoughtful."

Her mood changed and she replied, "seriously though, why don't you ask Dr. Merrick for some new pain medicine? There has to be hundreds of pain killers on the market, and I know one of them will help you."

"I know you are right, but it is my stomach that creates the problem. It's so sensitive, most medication make me sicker than I am. You know the old saying, *"Life sucks, and then you die.*"

Oh that's another peachy thought, Mom. Your on a roll today."

Aren't I though, I thought.

Again we changed the subject, and my thoughts immediately went to my mother. "Guess that I could blame my attitude on my morning talk with Myrtle May."

"That would do it," Rah replied.

"I gave her the news about my living with Brandon. It did not go over very well at all. I know that she realizes in her heart that it is the best thing for everyone, but you know how stubborn she can be."

"What was the outcome? Did she end up agreeing with your decision?"

"I think she did, but she says one thing, but truthfully she thinks and feels another way completely. She does realize that I am not going to change my mind. So, I have won the first battle, but probably not the war."

My hunger and anxiety took over, and I pleaded, "Rah, could we stop and get some coffee and a donut before I get to the doctors? If I eat a little more, I can take another pill. Today, I have to take

two pills. I hurt so bad, Rah."

Her answer was immediate, "I wish that I didn't feel so helpless Mom, is there anything I can do?"

"Yes, get me a donut," I said smiling.

"You are totally crazy."

"You never cease to amaze me, you never lose your sense of humor, "was her response.

"It's about all I have left, except for my hair," I said laughingly again. We pulled into the donut shop parking lot, and Rah ran in. She came out with my favorite, a chocolate covered glazed donut. I tried to eat it slowly, but it tasted so good. I know that I should have eaten it more slowly than I did, but what the heck. What was it going to do to me, make me sick?

"Here we are Mom."

"I am going over to Sue's this morning for a while. I'll just wait there until the tv cable company opens up."

"Don't worry, by the looks of all the cars in the parking lot, there are a lot of patients inside waiting. It's a sight to see Rah, all of us lined up in chairs, dressed in our little dressing gowns."

"Do you think that you will see Dr. Merrick this morning?"Rah asked.

"I am never sure. He is usually in the building but whether he will have me on his schedule, I won't know until I am in there. I hate the examination so much. It hurts me so badly. I would imagine that I have to be checked periodically. But, what do I know? I do as I am told." I looked at

her and advised, "You might as well leave now, Rah. I'll be fine. Remember, if I am not out when you return, come in and sit. I don't want you sitting out here in the cold."

"Alright, Mom," she agreed. "See you in a short while."

I was becoming accustomed to the daily routine of my treatments. I had gone into the locker room and undressed and was heading for the patients lounge when a nurse stopped me and asked me to follow her. It seemed that today was blood test day and the dreaded weigh in. I sat on the stool and the nurse took my blood pressure and removed two vials of blood. No problem there, I thought. *Here comes my worst nightmare, the scale. I stepped on to it holding my breath. 96 pounds was the recorded amount. "I gained a pound,"* I said proudly.

"Yes you did, congratulations," the nurse said smiling.

I entered the Patients Lounge smiling. I s aw Mrs. Peterson and she asked, "How you doing Honey?"

"Good, very good so far." I tried to use my most convincing positive sounding voice.

Surprisingly she said, "me too. I only have three treatments left.

"Then you're all done?" I asked.

"Well for this go round anyway. They will give me a rest for three months. Then the treatments

begin again. It gives the body the time it needs to recuperate."

"Oh, I understand," I replied.

A tall nurse came to the door and called my name out. " Ms. Ayer?"

"Yes, that's me."

"Dr. Merrick wishes to see you for a moment after your treatment this morning."

My heart sank. *Oh not another examination. Be brave, Pam. I was thankful that I had taken two pain pills this morning. I had a feeling that they were going to come in handy.*

I went into my treatment room and was greeted by the same two nurses that had been giving me my radiation. "I see you still have your hair," the taller nurse said.

I smiled and said, "Yes, so far so good."

"Come over here and let us take a look at your hair." she requested.

I walked over to them and I could feel them touching my hair. What exactly they were looking at, I was not sure. Perhaps there is a tell tale sign the shows if your hair is going to start to fall out.

"Little one, I don't think your going to lose it. Now if you will put your little self on the table, we can get this over with and you can go home."

The treatment was over quickly and I was on my way out when I turned and asked one of the nurses if she knew Dr Merrick's location.

"He is probably in his office," she said.

"I'll look there, because I was told me he wanted to talk to me before I left today." I knocked on his office door, and he was standing at the window with a file in his hand.

"Come on in," he said. He turned around and smiled. "Hello, Ms. Ayer. Already done with the treatment?"

"Yes, all set. The nurses are so nice to me. They checked my head and gave me their opinion regarding my hair."

"Yes, I noticed that you still have it. I don't think the chemo you are receiving will have an effect on your hair. It is a little early, but the hair usually starts to fall out immediately. So it does look promising. I asked you to see me this morning just to see how you were doing, and if you had any problems? "Are the morning appointment agreeable with you? Some people prefer the afternoon, but it is up to you."

"Oh no, the morning is fine for me."

"How are you feeling?"

"Well, I am really in pain. I wanted to ask you if there was another pill you could give me instead of the "*Motrin 800*" I am taking right now? It just doesn't seem to be taking the pain away any more."

"That is no problem, have you ever tried "*Tylenol*" with codeine?"

"No, I haven't."

"Well then, I will write you out a prescription and we will give it a try. You let me know, how you are reacting to it. If you should have any problems or reactions, just call here, and I will write out another prescription of something else. Anything else on your mind today?"

"No, that is it for today. I will see you tomorrow then. Oh Dr. Merrick, one more question, "How often do I have to have an internal exam?"I asked, making a face.

He hesitated, and then replied, "I know that they hurt you, but I have to do them on a regular basis to monitor what type of reaction your tumor is having to the treatments. As your tumor shrinks, so will the pain and discomfort, if that is any consolation to you."

"Yes, that helps a little," I said smiling weakly.

"Okay then, you go home and rest."

"I'll try doctor."

"Goodbye for now." I turned and walked out of his office.

When I got outside, Rah was not there. I considered going back into the building but changed my mind. The fresh air was no nice, even though it was very cold. I rested by leaning back on the building and waited. It wasn't long before I could see Rah's car coming down the road. I smiled, she is going to be upset to see me standing outside. Shall I tease her for being late? I think I shall.

Chapter 31
Price Tags

The next few days really flew by. The radiation treatments were completed for the week, and I was waiting for Rah and Brandon to come and pick me up at three o'clock. The recent days had been extremely difficult ones. My stomach had taken a serious turn for the worse, and accompanied with the discomfort of diarrhea, I had suddenly started to vomit every day as well.

My body was becoming extremely weak. If it were not for the drinks containing electrolytes, I don't believe that I would have been to stand up without losing my balance. Things were looking bad. I was not looking forward to what was ahead of me. How was I going to handle the furniture sale feeling so ill?

It had not occurred to me the furniture sale was scheduled for Halloween weekend. I had not checked the calendar when I placed my newspaper ad and, tonight was Halloween night. The little goblins should be completed with their trick or treating long before I am finished pricing my furniture. I don't think that the holiday will interfere with my plans very much. Perhaps an occasional interruption now and then by the candy seeking little children. Rah and Brandon had a time schedule today as well, and they were scheduled to bring their children out tonight in the search of candy in their neighborhoods as well. I told them," We will just get done what we have time for." Not to worry, I assured them. We can finish up tomorrow morning."

The whole family was going to be up in arms regarding my staying at my home alone tonight . But, I shall stand firm. I had asked Rah to stop at the local

K-Mart and a purchase some Halloween candy for me, and she assumed that it was for Nana's house. When she asked me why Nana wanted so much candy, I explained to her that it was for me. She used every logical reason in the book for me not to do such a thing.

"Staying alone? Are you insane Mom? she asked.

I looked at her and said, "Think about what you are saying? I have lived there for twenty six years, and for the passed two years, I have been totally alone. But lets not forget, during those two years, I have been very ill with the cancer growing inside me. I think that I can manage one more night in my own home alone. Halloween is special to me, I said defending my stand. I want to do this, and none of you can make me change my mind. If it will make you feel easier about it, bring the kids by this evening before you take them home. In that way, you can check on me. I will be fine, and I promise that I won't do anything foolish. I just need to be here, one more night."

She looked at me and could see that I was not going to back down on this subject. Okay Mom, but you can bet that you are going to see me and kids tonight," she said firmly.

"Good, I want to see them all dressed up. It wouldn't be the same if I didn't get the chance to see them." I smiled and said, "Then it's settled, right?" Rah said nothing. That was the way we left it. I did not want my mother to know about my plan. My mother thought that I would be returning

with Rah once the furniture was priced. I was going to leave it to Rah to advise my mother the news about my location for the night. I repeated to Rah, "Please, no more arguments about it."

Usually on Halloween, I would dress up and go with my grandchildren trick or treating. It had become a tradition for me as well as the kids. I enjoyed it so. I loved watching them get all dressed up. Usually they asked for my assistance for their make-up or what type of costume they were going to wear. They loved to see me in costume. One year I was a gangster, wearing a pin strike suit, hat, cigar and squirt gun. They loved that one. Another year I was *Elvira the Mistress of the Night,*" and who could ever forget my camouflage hunters outfit? We had so much fun together. Perhaps tonight I will surprise them and put on an old ugly bathrobe, curlers in my hair and cold cream on my face. That should scare the heck out them. But I will have to wait and see how I am feeling. There is a lot of work that has to be done. I hope my strength keeps up long enough to accomplish everything.

As a result of a telephone conversation earlier, it had been decided, that Brandon would take most of my clothes back to his home and hang them up in my new closet. He was not going to be very happy either when he heard that I was staying at my home, but he will have to deal with my decision.

Rah and Brandon arrived at almost the same time.

Rah asked, "Ready Mom?"

"Ready, let's get the show on the road," I said jokingly. We'll be back," was all I said to my Mom.

She smiled and said, "Don't work too hard Pam."

"I won't, I replied. I have my slaves with me."

On the way to my house we talked about tonight being Halloween and how the children were going to dress. It was supposed to be a big secret so that they could surprise me and make me guess who they were. I always guessed intentionally wrong, and that would always please them when they thought that they fooled me. I started the first serious conversation between us. "Well, you two know that this is going to be tough on all of us today. I don't mean the physical part . It's the emotional drain that we are going to feel preparing the furniture to be sold. This was your home as well as mine, and we had some wonderful times here," I said softly. A lump was already beginning to form in my throat. I told them, "I have prepared a list for both of you. It contains the prices I want placed on each item in the house. I did this last night, when I couldn't sleep, so if you see anything that you think is totally out of whack, let me know."

The ride lasted about fifteen minutes, and we drove down the long driveway leading to our home in total silence. Brandon broke the ice with, "The old homestead. We had some real good times here Mom, thanks to you," he commented.

"I didn't do it alone, your father worked hard as well."

Rah spoke up, "Oh please Mom, don't stick up for him. He was a lousy father, and never had time for any of us."

I interrupted her and said, "Your father was not a well man and you both know that. Half of what he did he was not responsible for. I have to say in his defense, he always worked. So lets drop the subject concerning him, and get moving on what we have to accomplish in only a few short hours."

As I unlocked the door and we entered the kitchen, I asked them, "Do you have your lists, paper, pens and tape?"

"Yes," Bran replied, "We do."

"Ready, set, go," I said. They were off in different directions in a split second. My job was to start cleaning out the refrigerator. When I opened the door, I found very little food. That's not uncommon for me, I thought. I have to leave something for me to eat tonight. I opened the freezer door and there were some tv dinners still there. Great, that will be my supper along with some candy.

I grabbed some garbage bags and began to clean out all the partially consumed jars of relish, mustard, old jelly, etc. Once that was done, I moved onto the cupboards. They were pretty close to empty as well. This job is not going to be as bad as I thought it would be. I had already decided to take only a few place settings and a few pots and pans to Brandon's house. I know that I am not going to need much, only enough for daily living and cooking.

The dining room was all set except for the hutch. It had been my ex mothers' in law dining room, and I did not want to sell her beautiful set of dishes. I thought to myself, *I will just give them to Rah, if she wants them. I want someone in the family to have them, not some stranger. I had loved my mother-in-law very much. She was a good woman and had always been very kind to me. I remember the last words she said to me before she passed away, "Please don't leave him, until I die." Can you imagine that? I did as she requested, but I stayed with him long after she had passed away. I had always hoped and prayed that someday he would change. But people don't change, especially when they are as seriously ill as he. Oh, I thought, I knew this was going to bring back a lot of memories that I had been suppressing this last year. Get on with it Pam, I scolded myself. Go to the next room and begin the work that has to be done.*

The bathroom was easy to clean out. I even had time to clean the shower and toilet with Clorox before I closed the door. On to the bedroom armed with garbage bags. I took one bag for what I wanted to keep and another for what was going to be thrown out. I started with the bureau drawers.

They were already pretty empty. I gave little thought of what I was doing and tried to sit on the bed while doing it. I moved on to the smaller dresser and did the same. If I had not worn it in a year, I was not going to wear now. That was the rule that I went by. Next, the closet. I pulled out all the clothes, sweaters, skirts, dresses all on hangers. One by one, I placed them on the bed. These Brandon could put right in his truck. All my perfume, lotions, and hygiene articles went into another smaller garbage bag. There, done. *"That didn't take long,"* I said to my self. *"It's kind of pitiful when you look at the entire picture." Everything that I possessed were in a few garbage bags."*

Brandon came down the stairs and said, "All priced Mom, except your bedroom furniture that is going to my house. I think that you could get a lot more money from the pool table, if you could find the right buyer."

"I know Brandon, but there's no time. We'll just take what we can get at this point."

"Dad would be furious, you know Mom," he replied frowning.

"Well the heck with him. If it wasn't for what he had done, I could have sold this house and made a lot of money. I am not going to worry about what he has to say about the pool table."

"He really screwed you, Mom, I am so sorry for what he did to you. Sorry for the way I put that, but it describes his actions perfectly."

"Oh, it's okay," Bran I said. Next came the pricing of the furniture on the porch.

Bran asked, "How is Rah making out downstairs?"

"Don't know, I haven't heard a peep out of her," I replied. I had no sooner got the words out of my mouth, when up the stairs she came.

"All done, Mom," she stated proudly. I even cleaned the bathroom and the kitchen while I was down there."

"Any questions on the pricing, Rah?"

"No, I think you are asking very fair prices, and I really think that everything will sell quickly."

"Great, then we are just about finished." I asked Bran, Would you go and get the clothes and bags in the bedroom and put them in your car? Don't take the bags in the hallway, as that stuff is going to the dump."

Rah suggested, "Do you want me to grab all your coats from the hall closets?"

"Please do Rah, I had forgotten all about them."

We were finished in record time. We took a break and I made some coffee. I had to throw away the milk, but we had some powered cream that sufficed.

Bran, I asked," I would like you to do one more thing for me, please get me some wood for the fireplace?"

He looked at me strange and then simply asked, "Why?"

"Because I am going to stay here tonight, that's why." Before he could open up his mouth, I said, "You are not going to stop me. I want to spend one last night in my own home. So son, just do as I ask this one time without giving me a problem. I have my medication, there is everything here that I need, so do not concern yourself about me staying here overnight. I want to sleep in my own bed one more time. So please, don't give me a hard time."

He looked at Rah and she just said, "Your not going to change her mind. I am going to bring the kids up tonight so that they can see her and trick or treat her, so why don't you bring up Alex and Bri. It will be just like the good old days."

Brandon got up from the table not saying a word and headed for outdoors. He was angry, I know, but he will deal with it. It only took a few minutes for Bran to bring in my logs. He placed them in the fireplace and then went to the kitchen and washed his hands.

"I am going to get the clothes now from the bedroom, give me a hand Rah."

"I will," she replied. It's getting late and we have to get home."

Once the clothes were in the car, we said our good-byes and I sent them on their way. I know that they were not happy campers (so the phrase goes) but this was something over which they had not control. I waved good-bye and watched them drive out of the driveway and turned to go back into my home.

Chapter 32

Halloween Night

As I walked through my kitchen, I began clearing off the kitchen table automatically and removing the dirty coffee cups that remained. I loaded them in the dishwasher only to discover that I had not done the load that remained there from the morning I had gone to the hospital. This is disgusting I thought to myself. You must have been feeling pretty lousy you left for work that day, as it was not like me to leave any work undone.

Lately, I had discovered that I seemed to be losing time. I think that it had to be the medicine I was on as I was not one to forget a lot of things. Every day seemed to be slipping away and all I could recall in my mind of what had actually occurred was tiny bits and pieces. Not a good thing.

I entered the living room and glanced at my phone. It was flashing, which could only mean I had messages. I pushed the button and the machine responded with, you have 37 new messages. I stood there for a moment contemplating whether or not to listen to them. *No, I thought to myself. Not right now. I just don't want to hear any of them. I was confident that it was mostly bill collectors, the bank, and a few well wishers from the Post Office. No, I can't handle any of them, not now anyway. Perhaps later on.*

I moved slowly over to the tv set, and picked up the remote, and clicked the button. Gee, I thought as the picture came on, the cable company hasn't shut me off yet. That's a pleasant surprise. Not there was ever anything interesting on all those channels, but it was the principal of the thing. My collection of VCR movies had grown through the years to almost 500 videos on tapes. I chose the movies that I wanted to see, and put the first tape in the machine. My choice was, of course, the movie "*Halloween*." I would watch the entire saga of "*Halloween*" tonight. That should cheer me up. It was beginning to get dark so I thought that I had better get the candy ready for the kids, should anyone come knocking. I just never knew how many kids would show up. It usually depended on the weather. Most of the kids in the neighborhood were grown up, just like mine,. But in the past few years, the parents had been driving the neighborhood children around to the different neighborhoods. I put the candy in several large bowls on the porch and turned on the outside lights. I do hope I see some little ones tonight. In the years past, I used to make Carmel apples for the kids. But in this day and age, apples are considered to be a dangerous item to receive from strangers. So I had to stop making them and went with the rest of the world and purchased wrapped candy.

I grabbed some newspaper and started to crumple it up, and headed for my fireplace. I was going to have the best fire tonight that I had ever made. And believe you me, when I say I can make a good fire, I really mean it. I loved my fireplace. It was about seven or eight feet in length, and made with beautiful flag stone. I was absolutely beautiful. Within minutes, the fire was going beautifully. I relaxed on the couch and started the movie "*Halloween*." I was only lying down for a few minutes when I became sick to my stomach. Oh please, not this, not now. I said out loud. I just want to have one good last night in my home. I was crying now. I ran for the bathroom, and lost whatever I had in my stomach, which I can assure you was not much, and returned exhausted to the couch.

I have to find out what is going on with this new development occurring with my stomach problem. I shall ask the first doctor I see, whether it is Dr. Johnson or Dr. Merrick. I am not particular which one at this point. I have to get a handle on this before it gets any further out of hand than it already has.

I dozed off quickly, suddenly I was awakened by the sound of the door bell. Startled, I almost fell off the couch. At first, I was very confused. For a few seconds, I was totally lost and had no idea where I was. As I slowly began to focus on the room, everything became familiar. I suddenly felt safe. I was home. I heard the door bell ring again. I hurriedly entered the kitchen and saw four smiling faces standing at the glass sliding door. I opened the door and heard four voices in unison yell, "Trick or Treat."

I tried to look very surprised and said, "Well, well, who do we have here?" I looked at the smallest of the group Kyle (name) and asked, "Is this little Johnny from next door?"

"No Meme, it's me, Kyle (name), he answered loudly.

"Oh Kyle, you dope, you told her who you are, now she knows it's us," Haley said disgustedly.

I couldn't help my self, and I started to laugh.

It was at that moment, Ra came in the porch door. "Did you guess it was them, Mom?"

"She didn't have to, stupid Kyle told her, " Tawnee admitted.

"That doesn't matter, I said. How did you do gathering candy at every ones house?"

They all smiled and lifted up their candy bags, which were filled to the very top.

"My goodness, you certainly have done well tonight."

"I still have all my candy, you are the only ones that came here tonight, so far. Why don't you help yourself."

Ra warned them, "Don't take it all just in case someone else does come. Meme has to have some candy left, just in case."

"Well come on in and let me inspect your costumes." Amanda had a pillow stuck in her shirt, which I thought was quite appropriate. She was still a child, and it broke my heart to think that she

was going to lose the precious childhood to which she was entitled., and become a mother at sixteen. Kyle (name) was a Power Ranger (his favorite), Tawnee was a witch and little Haley was a clown. I couldn't help but think how beautiful they all were.

We were are all headed for the living room when the door bell rang again. "I'll go and see who it is," I said to Rah.

"Go in and sit down with the kids, the fireplace is going and the movie *"Halloween"* is playing on the tv. "You might want to shut if off, so it doesn't scare the kids." I walked into the kitchen and there were two more little girls dressed as witches standing there.

"Trick or Treat Meme."

"Guess who we are" a little voice asked.

Of course I knew it was Alex and Bri, but I had to play the game.

"Is it Priscilla and Patty from the white house up the road?"

"No, guess again," a voice said giggling.

"Well I am going to have to give up. "Who are you? Do I know you?" I asked. Giggles, and more giggles.

"It's Alex, and Bri" a little voice said proudly. Alex had just gotten out the words, when Haley and Kyle (name) came running into the kitchen. For a moment it looked like a long lost family reunion. The kids acted like they had not seen each other for years, and then Brandon and Sue came into the kitchen at that moment. Their girls had made them hide on the porch while I was trying to guess who they were.

"How's it going Pam?" Sue asked.

"Good, it's going good. You and Rah are the only ones with trick or treaters who came here tonight. "Make sure Alex and Bri, get some candy. I have plenty left. I think it is too late for anyone else to come. Let's go in and join Rah in the living room and talk."

Brandon said proudly, "I told you that she would have the fireplace going."

"Of course," I replied.

"Are you feeling alright?" Sue asked.

"I am kind of tired. I am looking forward to a good nights sleep tonight."

"Well don't do any work, Mom, Brandon said quickly. Sue and I will be here early tomorrow morning."

Rah confirmed her appearance by adding, "I'll be here early also with Greg. So don't worry about anything tonight. Just go to bed and get some rest." Rah demanded.

They stayed for only a short visit, as they could see by my physical appearance, that I was totally exhausted and feeling very ill.

"Mom, I really hate leaving you here tonight." Rah said.

"Rah, I will be fine. If I need you the phone is still connected, I will call you. Now everyone go home, and stop worrying about me."

The kids were disappointed having to leave so fast, but letting them empty the candy bowls helped their mood. I hugged them all and kissed them good bye. I said, "I'll see you tomorrow morning." Goodbyes were said with long faces, and they were gone. As their headlights left the driveway, I could breath a sigh of relief. I just wanted to rest. I shut off the porch light and the kitchen lights and locked the doors. All I wanted now was to enjoy my fireplace, one more time.

I walked from room to room, trying to remember all the precious moments that each room held in my memory. I tried to convince myself that it did not matter if I could not physically visit these places, I shall have possession of them in my mind forever. The living room held memories of cooking marshmallows in the fireplace, and Christmas mornings. The kitchen table brought back memories of the little arguments of who was sitting next to me at the table. The boys bedroom brought a laugh out loud as I could picture Jason hiding in the closet because Brandon was singing the "Jaws" theme and scaring him. I actually had to calm him down and explain to Jay that sharks did not come into bedrooms. They were only in the salt water far out in the ocean.

Robin's bedroom brought back pictures of her girl friends staying over for a pajama party, and all the giggles, and whispering that went on until the sun came up. Even the bathroom held a special memory. I had held Brandon in my arms in the bathroom numerous times, as he fought for breath because of his bronchial condition. The shower spraying hot water, causing the room to be engulfed with steam. The steam assisting his ability to breath. I can recall being so scared, yet having to be so brave as not to scare him or the other children. I continued walking through each room, spending just long enough to recall a pleasant memory. I would not allow my thoughts to contain any negative reminiscent memories. So many happy memories. I shall treasure them always. No one, not the bank, nor anything else, no, not even this cancer can take them away from me. The saying goes, time heals all wounds. I wonder just how much time I have to heal? With that thought, I went to my bedroom and just climbed onto my bed. I did not even undress or get under the covers of the bed. I was just too tired and too heart sick. I closed my eyes, spoke to God and fell asleep.

Chapter 33
Get Ready

I wearily opened my eyes and glanced at my alarm clock. It was 5:00 a.m. I had slept almost the entire night, and it had been a very restful sleep, thank God, but upon waking, my pain was almost at the intolerable level. If I could just get to my pills, but they were in my purse which I had left in the living room. I stayed perfectly still, remaining in the same position in which I awakened in. My total concentration focused upon the ceiling fan that was humming above me. During the recent months I had taught myself how to concentrate on an object in a room until I reached an hypnotic state of mind. This dedicated type of concentration and breathing technique had enabled me to function through many difficult periods of pain. It was in this hypnotic state that I could physically leave the pain, and accomplish a task that seemed impossible. After several minutes of concentration, I was able to walk to the living room and retrieve the much needed medications from my purse.

I waited in the living room for the pills to take effect. I was fortunate to have left a glass of soda sitting on the coffee table, as I don't know if I could have gotten myself to the kitchen. *I asked the good Lord to help me today. Please give me the physical and mental strength to with stand the obstacles that were before me*, I prayed silently. There was so much work that had to be done. My kids were just going to have to handle most of it for me. What I had wanted to accomplish, upon waking, was both physically and mentally impossible for me to complete.

As soon as the pills had taken their full effect on my body, I returned to my bedroom. A pair of clean pants and sweatshirt were hanging in my clothes closet for today. I had deliberately left them hanging there. I took the clothes from the closet and made my way to the bathroom. I stripped and opened the shower door and stepped inside. The octagon window, which I had requested to be installed in the wall, still contained my favorite shampoo on the shelf. That was all it took for me to see to start me crying. I was in the shower, my own shower, for one last time. So many tears had been shed in this small cubical even before the diagnosis of cancer. This was my escape place. The tears began to fall almost immediately. Get them all out Pam. Let them flow. I kept thinking, today is going to be harder than fighting the cancer. I have to find the strength and ask God for his help in getting me through another difficult time in my life. I had to gain control. I could not allow any outbreaks of emotion in front strangers nor my own family.

I don't remember exactly how long I stayed in the shower. But I do know that I cried for a very long time. I think was skin was pretty wrinkled from being in water for that long of a period of time. But, my body sure was clean, and my hair was still on my head. I stepped out, dressed and went in the kitchen to make some coffee. I didn't have any bread or milk, so cereal and toast were out of the question. Perhaps the kids will think to bring some doughnuts with them when they arrive this morning. Until they get here the coffee will have to suffice.

I took my coffee and walked out to my sun porch as I had done for hundreds of mornings before leaving for work. I sat down on the wicker love seat and looked out the windows. It was a beautiful morning. Fall was such a lovely time of year. The leaves on the trees were gorgeous. It's so strange how your life can change in an instant. If only….How many times have I said that lately? If only I had done so many things differently. Would I have had the intelligence to do things differently? Who knows? If only…?

I sat there sipping the coffee and just looking out into the orchard. I saw something move just beyond the first row of apple trees. There it was, a deer. A huge deer. A smile crossed my face as I remembered the time my ex was bringing the boys on a deer hunting trip to upstate NY. I recall standing on the porch, waving good bye to them as they drove out of the driveway. I had contained my laughter all the time I was waving good bye. There it stood, not 25 feet away from them. A huge deer with a full set of antlers just watching them. It was as if he were laughing as well. I stood and watched that deer for over an half an hour. He just walked around the orchard and ate leisurely without a care in the world. After all, the great hunters had left the area. Just another great memory that I shall treasure.

I was still smiling when Brandon's car pulled into the driveway. I opened the porch door and said, "My goodness, you are here early."

"We've got a lot to do," Brandon replied. Sue had already gotten out of the car and was pulling large cardboard signs out from the backseat of the car.

"Oh great," I said. "You remembered to make the signs."

Brandon gave me one of his smirks and simply replied, "Of course Mother dear."

I smiled and thought to myself, put aside the old memories start making new ones Pam. Today is going to be one memory for the book. It is time to move on. My new life awaits me, I must therefore get past today in order to face tomorrow.

Sue handed the signs to Brandon and started walking towards the house. She stopped just before entering the porch. "I forgot something in the car," she said. She turned and ran in the direction of the car. I *started walking toward the living room and thought to myself, oh to be so young and have so much energy.* I sat down in the living room still holding my coffee cup which was almost ready for a refill, when Sue entered the room. She was holding in her hands a box of doughnuts. "For you, Pam" she said smiling. We all love you."

I got up and walked over to her and put my arms around her. "Thanks for being here, I said. You will never know how much I appreciate what you and Brandon are doing for me. Don't give it a second thought, she replied. With everything that you have done for everyone in this family it is the least that we can do in return."

We brought the doughnuts back into the kitchen, and Sue started to make another pot of coffee. Brandon had returned and said, "The signs are put up. I put one on the telephone pole down the road, another out in front of the house, and the third one next to the Apple orchard sign."

"Thanks, Sonny boy," was my reply. Where are the girls this morning?" I asked.

"Oh they stayed over at my mothers house last night when we returned from Trick or Treating. They send their love."

"Tell your Mom when you see her I said thank you. It is very kind of her to watch them today." Sue replied, "My mother wanted me to tell you, if there is anything that she can do, just let her know."

"What's next, Mom?" Brandon asked.

"I want you to put anything that is not too heavy out in the lower area of the driveway. Things like lamps, small tables, and book cases. Brandon, I am leaving it up to you today to run the show. I am too sick to do much, I afraid that I can't be much help."

Sue walked over to me and put her arm around me. "Okay, that's enough, your going back to bed. "You can hardly stand up. Come on, lets go right now."

I started to argue, when the porch door opened and in walked Greg and Rah. "Hello, is anybody up?" Rah yelled.

"We're in the living room," Brandon called out.

"What's going on?" Rah asked as she walked into the room.

"We are trying to Mom to go back to bed and lie down. She is sick as a dog," Brandon replied. Before I could say another a thing I had to run into the bathroom, I was going to be sick again.

By the time I returned to the living room, Jay and Ann were sitting with the rest of the family group.

"Mom, just turn around and go back to the bedroom and get some rest, even if it is for only an hour or two," Jay said pleadingly.

"I am afraid that I have no choice, I answered. Even if I wanted to help, and I do, I just can't, " I admitted.

Rah spoke up next, "Mom, we are going to handle everything. We will get you, if we encounter any problems. You need to rest. Come on Mom, right now." She stood up along with Sue and Ann. They walked toward me with serious concern on their faces.

"Okay, I am going I have faith in all of you. Do the best you can and try and make me some money." I walked with the three girls to my bedroom door. I can take it from here. Go and help your husbands."

Rah asked, "Mom do you want me to shut the bedroom door?"

"Yes, I don't want strangers to see me in bed," I said laughing.

Rah smiled, "No we can't have that." With that final statement she gently closed the door.

Chapter 34
Going, Going, Gone

Oh good Lord, it's 2:30 in the afternoon! I couldn't believe my eyes when I saw the time on my alarm clock. Should I go out into the living room and see what was happening? Do I have the courage to go and look and see strangers walking around in my house? My mind was racing with questions. I tried to listen for voices, but I could hear nothing with my bedroom door shut. "It's now or never," I said out loud. I sat up and waited for the wave of nausea to strike, but nothing happened. The pain had returned, so the discomfort from that forced me to move. I needed another pill. I guess there is no escaping the inevitable. Don't forget to take another "Xanax," Pam, I said to myself. I have a feeling that your going to need it.

I slowly opened my bedroom door and walked out into the hallway. I could hear conversations coming from the kitchen area, and some commotion going on as well. I was so afraid to look, but I had too. I forced myself to walk down the hall further. The first person I saw was my son Jay. He was holding a lamp in his hands. He gave me a weak smile and said, "Hi Mom." I returned his smile and kept walking toward him. The shock that was about to hit me is indescribable. There was nothing in the living room except my tv and my collection of movies. Everything else was gone, even the curtains. The shock had to have registered on my face, as Jay motioned for me to go back to my room. "No," I said, "I have to see, I have to face it." I kept my feet moving and turned into the dining room. Or should I say what used to be the dining room. It too was totally empty. Even the blinds on the windows were missing. In a trance I kept moving. In the kitchen again then was nothing. No refrigerator, stove or kitchen set. The dishwasher was still there, but I presume the reason for that was it was built in to the cupboard. My patio furniture was being loaded into a large grey pick-up truck by Brandon and Greg. I could see Rah and Sue in the driveway talking to some strangers. I felt extremely weak in my legs and I leaned over the kitchen sink to splash some water on my face. I filled a glass of water and took the pills which I had been carrying around in my hand. I couldn't get the medication in me fast enough. The room started to spin and I thought, *oh no, I am going to pass out. I wanted to cry out, God help me. But nothing came out of my mouth. I turned and grabbed for the downstairs basement apartment door knob. I had to get to a place, where I could see nothing of what was going on. I opened the door and began my descent, holding on to the rail for my very life.*

Ann was just approaching the bottom of the stairs and saw me. "Pam, what are you doing?' she asked frantically.

I had to come down here to get away from everything going on out there.

"I know, she said. I can't believe it myself. I have never seen so many people. One man bought all the furniture down here. He must own a second hand store somewhere. He wanted everything. Jay and Greg helped him load everything on his huge truck he brought here."

"What is left upstairs?" I asked weakly.

"Only your wicker bedroom set. The pool table is still up there, but a man paid for it. Brandon and Jay have to dismantle it tonight. The man is returning tomorrow with some people to take it away. I slumped down on the stairs, not able to stand any longer. My legs felt like pure rubber (and that is a true statement) "Pam, you should go back to your bedroom, if this is getting to you. You made a lot of money, if that is any consolation for you," she said tenderly. She reached over and touched my shoulder. "Are you alright?" Ann asked.

"I will be fine, Ann, I just need some time alone, Please, " I begged.

"Do you want me to leave you here on the stairs?" she asked.

"Please, Ann," I replied. "I would appreciate it."

"Okay, but if you need anyone, you just yell," and she touched my shoulder again and headed back up the stairs.

I sat there for only a moment. I had to gather up my strength for my walk through of the basement apartment. It took a moment or two and I got my legs to move. Nothing was there, even the washer and dryer were gone. My God, how hard my kids must have worked. Then a feeling of panic struck me, and I had to get out. I ran for the back door of the apartment. I ran and ran for the first apple tree that I could get too. I sat down and began crying. Crying, sobbing, and gasping. I cried so hard that I could not breath. I am not sure whether it was a panic attack or just reality hitting my body. But I must have lost consciousness. For the first time in my life I had submitted totally to the devastation of my life. I am not sure how long I lay there before the children found me. I could hear Rah's voice, "Mom, Mom?" I opened my eyes and the first face I saw was my beautiful daughter Rah. Everyone else was standing around with a look of fear and terror in their eyes.

"Mom, Mom, talk to me," Rah repeated.

I looked at her and said simply "Hi Rah. What happened?" I asked.

"You scared us to death, that is what happened," she stated with her voice shaking. None of us could find you, Ann spotted you under the tree.

" Why did you come out here, Mom?" Brandon asked.

"I felt that I had to get away from it all. I'm sorry, it was just to much for me to take, I confessed.

I didn't want to cry in front of all those strangers. I would have felt like some kind of a nut."

Rah and Greg reached down and help me to stand up. Brandon and Jay each took one of my arms and guided me toward the house. "I feel so stupid," I confessed. Their concern for me was so touching. My heart was so full of love for all of them. What a family I have, I am a lucky woman, I thought to myself. "To hell with the furniture. What I have money can't buy," I said out loud to all of them.

We all returned to the living room, or what was left of it. "You guys must be one terrific bunch of sales people, that is all I can say." I said smiling.

Brandon said, "Mom, Rah is going to take you to Nana's to get away from all this. We have all discussed this, and this is the way it is going to be even if we have to throw you in the car." The rest of them echoed their agreement.

"Alright, I know your right, I admitted. Let me get my purse first. My medication is in it, and I desperately need it."

I got into Rah' s car and waved at my sales crew. Rah and I were once on the road again. "Mom you really did do very well with the sale of everything. You should have plenty of money to have Brandon fix you a beautiful apartment. So stop your worrying," she pleaded.

"Was there any trouble at all with the customers?"

"No, not with the customers, but Jay and Brandon almost got into it regarding who was holding onto the money for each sale. But I will admit that they settled it between themselves without any scene and everything went smoothly from there. Brandon has the money, in case you want to know," she said reassuringly. Brandon, Greg and Jay are planning to bring your bedroom set, the white one, over to Brandon's house so that you can sleep there tonight. I want you to stay there tomorrow and do nothing but rest, she ordered. You really did scare the hell right out of all of us today. We thought we had lost you," she started to cry.

"Oh don't cry Rah, I am alright," I admitted.

"Well you just remember what Monday holds for you, more Chemo. So I really mean it Mom, tomorrow you rest and we will finish up at the house. I gave Nana a call before we left and she is cooking you some soup for dinner."

"Oh no," I teased. "Not her beef stew?"

Rah had to smile at that statement. "I hope not for your sake, your stomach could not handle that right now." We both started laughing.

"Just promise me that you won't worry." Rah pleaded.

"Rah, I am not worried anymore. Afer how you kids handled today, I have total confidence in you. "I am so proud of all of you, I said emphatically. When you get back to the house, please tell them all that I love them and I thank them from the bottom of my heart."

"I will Mom, she said grabbing my hand and squeezing it. I will Mom, I promise."

Rah dropped me off at my mothers. "You stay seated, I can get in the door by myself, I assured her. Just wait until I open the door and get in, then you can leave. Just in case," I said teasingly. Rah smiled and I opened the car door and stepped out.

Chapter 35

A New Start

My Mom and Dad were standing at their door when I walked in. My Mom practically grabbed me and yanked me inside of her apartment. "Are you alright ? Rah told me what happened to you, she said they found you on the ground under one of the apple trees in the yard," she exclaimed. I sat down in Dad's recliner and proceeded to try and explain to her just what the circumstances were that had caused me to be in that predicament. I went through the entire day, explaining that I had slept through most of the confusion and that the total shock of seeing everything I owned gone caused me to pass out.

"The kids did a wonderful job. They took over and handled the entire situation, working together to accomplish the extremely difficult job of selling my possessions," I explained.

My father asked, "How much furniture is left?"

"Almost nothing. The pool table is still there only because Brandon and Jay have to disassemble it either tonight or tomorrow so that it can be removed from upstairs. A man who owned a bar somewhere is Providence bought it, and he is returning tomorrow with a truck to take it away.

I am not sure if my pine bedroom set was sold, because I was sleeping in it for most of the day. Of course they could have sold it once I left the house, I said. I just don't know at this point."

My mother emphatically stated, "Your not going back there tomorrow."

"This time I agree with you Mom. " The look on her face from me agreeing with her was quite amusing.

"You mean to say, that you're not going to argue with me on this?" she asked.

"No, I am not. I have had enough, and I said my good byes to my home last night. I think it's best if I never step foot in the house again, and the kids agree with me."

"Mom, I am kind of hungry and Rah told me you said you had made some soup. Do you have any left?"

"There is plenty of it left in the kitchen. she said. It's chicken soup. Lets go out there so you can sit and put some food in your stomach. Rah told me that all you have had to eat is doughnuts and coffee for the entire day. No wonder you passed out, especially in your weakened condition," she said in her most disgusted tone of voice.

Ra and I have always had a private joke regarding my mothers ability to cook soup. I have never meant to hurt her feelings, but whenever she made soup I could not pass up the opportunity to tease her about it. The truth is Mom is always so serious, that's where the fun lies. Her sense of humor has always been very slim. Therefore whenever the opportunity arose to give her a little jab of some sort, I very seldom missed my chance to get in a little bitty jab, and right now was no exception to the rule.

When she placed the bowl of soup in front of me I had to say some little thing just to get her going. "My, my, mother, you know just how much I love your soup. It is always so tasty and delicious," I said smirking.

"Don't you even start on my soup, Pam. Just be quiet and eat every bit of it," she demanded. But I did see a slight smile cross her face. But I want to be honest here, the soup did taste good, and I was so hungry by this point. So I made my mother happy, and my hungry body happy by finishing the entire bowl of chicken soup.

Time for my medication, I thought. *I don't want to be in any pain when Brandon comes to pick me up for the trip to his home.*

My mother must have been reading my thoughts and said, "Why don't you just stay here tonight?"

"No, Brandon is going through a lot of trouble for me moving my bedroom furniture on top of everything else that was done today. It's the least I can do for him in return. Besides I am looking forward to getting settled in my new apartment," I said smiling. "It is a lot more comfortable then your couch Mom, no offense."

She gave me one of her special looks and raised her eye brows, " I can understand that, but what is happening tomorrow?"

"As far as I know all, of the kids are going up to the house and finish up everything. I really don't think that there will be many more people showing up for the sale, and even if there are a few stragglers, there's not much left to sell. Rah told me when she dropped me off, that she was going to be packing up all my odds and ends, such as linen, dishes, towels and whatever else they could find that I will need for my new apartment. There is no need for me to have to purchase all those necessary items when I already have them."

My mother sat there for a moment and then asked the inevitable question, "How much money did you make from the sale?"

"I have no idea what so ever. All I know right now is what the kids keep telling met was that I had made enough money to do what I wanted in regards to my new apartment. So I just left it at that. I will be so happy when all of this is over. It will give me one less thing to worry about," I replied. "I am taking one step at a time, for right now. That is all I can do, or I will make my self crazy. You can understand that, can't you Mom?" She answered with me a nod.

Brandon and Sue arrived at almost nine o'clock. He looked exhausted. "Do you want something to eat?" I asked both of them. "Maybe a cup of coffee?"

Brandon replied, "No thanks, we had a pizza at our house when we brought your furniture over there." Are you ready to leave?" he asked.

"Yes, I am. Let's go so you can get home and get some rest." I told my mother that I would call her tomorrow, and we grabbed our coats and left.

There was nothing said between us until I got into the car. Brandon handed me the piece of paper I had given him with all the prices that I wanted for each piece of furniture. He had carefully placed a check mark next to each item that was sold. On the bottom of the sheet of paper was the total figure of the entire sale. I was amazed. "You got exactly what I asked for on each piece?" I asked.

"Yes, we did. We stuck to the prices to the letter. There were so many people there, that if someone did not want to pay your price, someone else did. So, it worked out perfectly."

"Brandon," I asked, do you think we have enough to complete the apartment?"

"According to my figures, Mom, it's pretty damn close. You should be able to have the apartment of your dreams," he said with total confidence in his voice.

We stopped and picked up Alex and Bri at Sue's mothers house, before going to Brandon's. They came running out the door, all smiles, eager to give me hugs and kisses. They were so excited about me living with them. I was hoping and praying that this would work out for all of us.

When Brandon put his key in the door, he turned and said, "Mom, if you don't like the way the furniture is arranged just tell me. I'll place it any way that will meet your approval." We were all so excited. We walked through the framed rooms and came to my new bedroom. The door was closed.

Brandon put is hand on the door knob and opened the door. I was stunned. The room looked as though it had come from a magazine picture. A beautiful powder blue rug was on the floor, the walls were painted a very light blue on the top, and dividing the walls was a rustic paneling on the bottom. Everything was placed perfectly. New curtains were hung on the windows and a matching bedspread on the bed itself. All my perfume, lotions, jewelry box and other personal items were carefully arranged on the dressers. There were no words that I could say to express how I felt. All I could do was sit on the bed and cry. Alex and Bri quickly came and sat next to me, one on each side. "Do you like it Meme?" Alex asked.

"Like it, I love it. Son, when did you have time to do all of this?" I asked, still crying.

"It was all here, Sue picked out everything with the girls." he said proudly. It was just waiting for the bedroom set to arrive. It only took us about a hour to complete all the little extras."

"You really do like it?" Sue asked.

"I have no words to express my feelings, I can only say thank you," I answered, still crying.

"Mom, there only one problem," Brandon said.

I looked up at him with tears in my eyes, "What?"

"I forgot to put in a heat vent, so you will have to freeze to death this winter." I busted out into laughter, and so did everyone else.

"I"ll fix it Mom, so don't worry," Brandon replied still laughing.

At that point we decided that it was time for a good cup of coffee and walked upstairs. "There is still some work to do at the house, Mom. But, we should be able to finish up totally tomorrow by noon. So, I don't want you to worry about the house anymore. It's all going to work out. You are here now, and we will take care of you from now on."

Sue asked, "Pam have you taken your medication?"

"Yes, I took it while I was at my mothers."

"Well I want you to take a container of water with you downstairs before you go to bed. That is so you won't have to walk up the stairs if you get thirsty in the middle of the night."

"That's a good idea Sue, I'll do that."

"Also, if you need anything at all, just tap on the walls, our bedroom is right above you and we can hear you easily. Promise me that you will do that Pam?" Sue pleaded.

"I will, so stop worrying."

"Monday I will start on the bathroom for you. I should be able to finish it in a day or two at the very most. All the connections and pipes are there, it will be no problem at all for me. I know you Mom, so don't concern yourself about that problem. Now lets all turn in and get some sleep. Tomorrow is going to be here fast, and there is still work to do, and today has been a long day for everyone," Brandon stated.

Chapter 36
Breathe a Sigh of Relief

The sounds from the road in front of Brandon's house were very different than any sounds I have been used to hearing in the morning. My son's house was set back from the road, but it was a main road in the town of Fairfield, which meant traffic and a lot of it. I just relaxed and watched the ceiling fan that Brandon had installed go round and round. I was used to a ceiling fan, so I found it comforting. I had discovered last night that Brandon had even installed a cable line for my tv. He had even thought of a telephone extension for my room. He had thought of everything. I was so proud of him. I laid there feeling pretty good. Not much pain and there had been no feelings of nausea. So far so good, I thought.

I had slept well with no bathroom trips. Which helped me considerably, as I didn't want to have to go up and down the stairs in the middle of the night. I had figured that if that problem had developed, I would simply spend the rest of the night on the living room couch. I had no idea what time it was. I had not bothered to set the alarm clock sitting on my night stand before I fell asleep. It can't be very late because I don't hear any movement coming from upstairs. I don't think anyone has gotten up yet. I sat up in the bed as I suddenly heard voices coming from outside. "Car Wash, come get your car washed" were the words I heard. "What the devil," I said right out loud. I got out of the bed and walked to my window. I could hear the voices but I was unable to see anyone from the position of my windows. I took my robe, that Sue had placed, on my vanity chair and swung it around my shoulders. I'll just take a walk upstairs and see what is going on. I climbed the stairs slowly, still hearing no sounds from the upper part of the house. Only the voices from outside.

When I reached the top of the stairs, I saw the kitchen table set very neatly with boxes of cereal, a glass or orange juice, an empty bowl and a coffee cup. I looked to my left and saw two little girls all smiles.

"Good morning Meme," they both yelled. We made you breakfast, Alex confessed proudly. Mommy and Daddy have already left for your house."

"Well how very nice of both of you,"I replied. Can you tell me what all the yelling is about outside?"

Bri replied, "Oh that, it's just the high school kids raising money for uniforms. They do that every Sunday."

"Well, isn't that special, especially so early in the morning."

Alex looked at me strangely, "Meme, it's not early. It's almost 11:30."

"Oh, my goodness," I said shocked. I slept that late."

"Yep you did, and we were very quiet, "Bri said proudly.

"I'll say you were, I didn't hear a peep out of you two." They both smiled on that statement.

"Are you ready for coffee?" Alex asked. Mom has it all set to go for you, I just have to turn it on."

"Why thank you Alex, yes I could sure use a cup of coffee.

" What about your pills Meme?" Bri asked.

"Oh yes, I had better take them, but my purse is downstairs."

"No problem, I'll go and get it." and off Bri ran to get my purse.

I asked Alex, "What time did Mommy and Daddy leave this morning?"

"About 7:30," she replied.

They must have been tired, I thought.

"Mommy said "She didn't think they would be long today, and that we are supposed to take care of you."

Well you two are certainly doing a very good job, and I thank you both." I finished my breakfast, (some kind of fruity stuff) and we decided that we would sit on the couch and talk. They are such intelligent little girls, so caring and loving. We watched tv until I had to make my trip to the bathroom.

" I have to take a shower girls, can you show me where the towels are?"I asked. They both jumped up and were headed for the bathroom.

"We'll get you everything that you need. We know where everything is so you wait until we say okay, okay?"

"I'll just sit right here until you tell me," I replied chuckling. A few minutes passed and I could hear them talking to each other and then I got the okay.

"Okay Meme, it's all ready for you," Alex's yelled.

"I'm be right there, " I answered. I got up off the couch and headed for the bathroom. The two little ones had everything lined up. Shampoo, soap, conditioner, towels and face cloths. "Thank you sweethearts, I can manage now." They smiled and left the bathroom and shut the door as they were leaving. I know one thing this morning, there shall be no tears in this shower, not today.

It was a little after three when Brandon and Susan arrived back home. I watched from the front room window as they removed garbage bag after garbage bag from the car. Alex opened the front door asking them if they needed any help. "No, you go take care of Meme, we can handle this," her father replied. When everything was brought into the house, they both came up stairs and collapsed on the couch.

"All done Mom, the only few things remaining are your movies and a few other small things laying around." Brandon said proudly. I will get the remaining stuff one night this week on my way home from work." I reached over and gave him a hug. I know he hates it when I do that, but I had to show my appreciation in some way and the words wouldn't come.

"Thank you Sue, as well."

"We couldn't have done it without all the help we had. Jay and Ann, plus Rah and Greg."

Brandon was proud to say this, "For once we all worked together like a family. No arguing at all Mom. You would have been proud."

I looked at my son, with tears in my eyes and simply said, "I have never been prouder of any of you than I am today. I will call everyone a little later on and thank them personally," I confessed.

Sue quickly got in the conversation, "If I don't tell you now I will forget, Rah is coming after you tomorrow morning at 7:30. She said be ready, or you will be in big trouble.

I smiled, "I'll be ready, she is a lot bigger than me, I can't mess with her anymore."

Brandon seemed a little concerned, "Were the girls good?"

Sue asked, "Did they feed you? I told them to."

"Oh my goodness yes. They waited on me all day," I confessed

Alex quickly added, "I gave Meme a sandwich for lunch. I made her a ham and cheese on toast."

Bri had to get in her say, "I gave her potato chips and a pickle."

"Yes, they did, the meal was delicious," and I gave them a hug right then and there. I love you both so very much." I confessed.

"We love you too." they both echoed.

We five sat and talked all evening until almost 11 p.m. "I had better get to bed, as I know the morning is going to come fast. I have already taken my pills, so I will say goodnight." I turned to say something more, but the darn old lump in my throat was becoming bothersome, so I just turned and headed for the stairway without saying anything more.

Chapter 37
Chemotherapy....Repeat Performance

Rah arrived a earlier than I had anticipated. Apparently she had been able to get the kids up and moving more in advance than normal this morning. We used the extra time to relax with Sue, and enjoy another cup of coffee before the dreaded treatments that I had to face today. I hated doing both of them

on the same day. I am thankful though; I only have the double dose once a week. Some of the suffering women that I have seen have to do it almost every day. How they can withstand this physical torture is far from my comprehension?

Sue had been trying to convince Bri all morning to wear a particular outfit to school. Bri, as usual was determined to wear another. I know that Bri is young, but let me say this; she has the determination of a adult women. God Bless the man that marries her and attempts to change her mind regarding something. Good Luck! It was quite amusing to watch. I can say that because I have been there and done that, as the saying goes. As a matter of fact, it was with Bris' dad. Yes, good old dependable Brandon. Stubborn as a mule. I usually won out, but he never went down without a fight, and I know that

Rah had been in the same difficulty with little Miss Amanda. I looked at Rah, when Sue and Bri were arguing, and I tried very hard not to laugh.

"Does this bring back any memories for you, Rah?" I asked smiling.

"Oh my God yes," she said. "Amanda was worse than Bri. Do you remember how she would wear a second set of clothing under what I made her wear to school, Mom? Yes, I remember very well."

Then Sue added, " Well Bri had better not try that one, or her father will hear about it. He won't tolerate that type of behavior, even if she is his little Princess.

"Kids are much more difficult now than when I was younger." I commented.

"Oh how many times have I heard that one?" Rah said laughing. But in all honesty, I think you are right, Mom. I am beginning to have trouble with Tawnee and her little attitude as well. She is developing physically, and she is already attracting the boys.

I had to excuse my self from the table, another bathroom trip. The nausea and vomiting had arrived for another return engagement. The nausea had visited once before in the early hours, around 5 :00 a.m. and has now returned for an unwanted encore.

"Mom, we must speak with the doctors about this! You are getting worse and getting thinner and thinner."

"I know, Rah. I'll promise I will tell someone today about the problem."

"Good, you better or I will," Rah said defiantly.

"It just takes every bit of strength out of me. It doesn't even matter what I eat, anything does it to me. Maybe I have an ulcer or colitis?"

"Maybe, but we won't know until we ask someone, will we?"

"Okay Rah, I get the point." I said giving in.

"Pam, you are much too trusting of a person," Sue replied. "You need to ask more questions."

I admitted that I should find out more about my disease, but I did not go into the details of my desire to know where I got this cancer with Rah and Sue at this time.

Rah turned to Sue and said, "I'll bring her home when she is finished with the radiation treatments. It should be somewhere around 2:30p.m. or 3:00p.m."

"That's fine Rah, I'll be here and I will have a key made for you today Pam when I am out and about."

"Great idea, I hadn't even thought of that," I confessed.

"Come on Mom, time to get out butts moving," Rah said teasing.

"Oh, I rather that you didn't put it that way," I said smiling.

"Funny Ma, really funny, lets leave, how"s that? Better?" Rah asked.

I just looked at her and smiled.

As we were starting to walk down the stairway, Rah turned to Sue and asked, "Don't you agree that it is a good idea for Mom to stay at my house over the weekend, and then on Monday afternoon she can return here and stay until Friday afternoon? Then she will be with me for Monday morning Chemotherapy treatments."

Sounds great to me," Sue answered. Is that okay with you Pam?

"Anything you two decide is fine with me." Rah and I continued out the door and got in the car and headed for Providence.

"You know Mom, that will really work well. Brandon will be able to work on the apartment all weekend, and you won't have to be disturbed while he is doing it."

"Actually, it is better for Brandon, that way and I won't be in his way," I admitted.

"You said that Mom, not me," Rah said wearing a huge grin.

While we were driving, Rah suggested we find out a little more information on how long the treatments were going to take. One month, two months? "Let's just try and get them to give us some kind of time frame."

"We can try," I answered. But both the doctors seemed very evasive every time I asked. I think it is because they really don't know themselves. I should be thankful that they even hint that they are going to kill this tumor. That is a lot more than some of these women have heard.

Of course there was a lot of traffic heading for Providence. Rhode Island may be small, but there is a lot of people on the roads at eight o'clock in the morning. All of them going are going to work, and mostly in Providence or Fairfield. But good old Rah, she knows here way around. She took so many side streets, she had me totally lost and nervous. We were driving through such a bad neighborhood, I almost had a heart attack. But, Rah got me there in record time, plus safe and sound.

"I hope that this treatment goes as well as last week, " I confessed.

"It will Mom, it will,"she said positively.

"At least I am not scared to death, and know what to expect."

"You have got that in your corner, and keep those positive thoughts."

We walked into the building and headed directly for the lab. My blood was drawn quickly and painlessly. We returned to the lobby and entered the elevator. I thought to myself, I am really getting good at this. There was a time in my life, (panic attack time) when an elevator would have been out of the question, no matter how many stairs were ahead of me.

The door opened and, I gave my name to the girl at the desk. I noticed that she was someone I had not seen before, and we were told to sit in the waiting room. That I didn't mind at all. I truly enjoyed the beauty of the room. I was hopeful that I would see the young girl again, but again she was no where in sight.

"Ms Ayer," the nurse called.

"Right here. " We both stood up and began following the nurse in the direction of a treatment room. It turned out to be the same room that I had last week. *Familiar territory*, I thought. *That's a good thing.* One of the nurses that treated me last week entered the room with a big smile on her face. "Good morning, Ms. Ayer," She said. "What lovely hair you have," all the while smiling.

I returned her smile and said, "So far so good, looks like you were correct."

"You will know much more by tomorrow morning. If nothing occurs from today's treatment, you will have it made. Don't buy a wig yet," she said smiling. "Now which hand did we use last week? Oh I can tell, I still see the battle marks. Seriously, how are you doing? she asked. We have a few minutes before the blood test are available, so we can talk. Did you have any side effects from the Chemo?"

"I really don't think so, I said. The only problem I have is with my stomach. I have so much trouble with having to run to the bathroom, and now I am vomiting all the time, I confessed. Do you think I will see the doctor today, because I really need some medication to slow this vomiting down."

She looked at me strangely, and then asked "Did you not get a prescription from the doctor for side effects? What you are describing to me are the effects of the Chemo and radiation treatments."

"They are?" I asked stupidly.

"Yes, most definitely!" I could tell that the nurse was very upset. "You should have been given something last week to totally prevent this! "I will be right back." She stormed out of the room.

"Looks like someone is in trouble," Rah said.

"Oh I hope not."

"I just want to begin feeling a little better than I have been. I expect to feel lousy with all these treatments, but I don't have the knowledge to know exactly what to expect."

I sat and waited for the results of the blood test. While I was sitting there, I made a promise to myself to look up information regarding this disease. Now that I am at Brandon's house, Sue will take me to the library and I can retrieve some answers to my many haunting questions.

Just a few minutes passed when another nurse came in and asked, "Are you all set to be connected?"

"Yes, I am, " I replied softly. Once again, the nurse knew exactly what she was doing. I felt just a slight pin prick,. My medicine was brought in with my name on each of the three bags. The nurse hooked the IV to the bags and the machine started to click. After a half hour passed, I was asked if I was hungry. Today, I said yes. I was brought a bowl of oatmeal, toast and orange juice. They even brought Rah some coffee, lucky bugger. No coffee for me. I'll just wait until we are on our way to the radiation doctors and then I will get a large cup of coffee. I was being very smug and resentful. I love coffee as I have stated before. *Forgive me God, for being such a spoiled brat. I promised myself to be more patient and understanding.*

"You know Rah, you could just drop me off next Monday rather than wait around here for hours. There is nothing here for you to do."

"Not on your life, Mom," she said without flinching. I am staying right with you. Don't suggest that again, cause I am not paying any attention to you if you are going to make stupid suggestions like that."

The subject was quickly changed and we sat there and talked about yesterdays furniture sale. She told me about all the people that came. Some of the people were from the Post office. Whether they were there to buy or to try and find out information in anyone's guess, but Rah did admit there were some strange characters out and about. She admitted that her, Sue, and Ann had done a lot of giggling as regards to the people and how they acted.

"Greg didn't hurt his back did he, doing all the lifting and moving?" Greg has always had back problems and yesterday I know that he had really put his back through hell.

"No Mom, and don't worry about Greg. Jay and Brandon were there every time to help him. He was fine last night and this morning."

"That's good, I was concerned that he would hurt himself and put you two in more of a financial pickle then your currently facing." We were still talking about Greg when the "angry" nurse came back into the room. She was holding a prescription for me.

"I found Dr. Johnson and advised him of your symptoms. This medicine should help you a great deal. I only wish that you would have called earlier; we could have helped you sooner with the side effects."

"Oh, that's okay, I should have asked." I admitted.

The nurse quickly replied, "No that's not your responsibility. It's the doctors. But the situation has been handled now. She winked at me, gave me the prescription and left the room. "Now there is a considerate person," Rah commented

"You are right there Rah."

The IV continued to drip for another half hour or so. We sat and watched some tv talk show. Rah got to laughing, and said, "Mom, I think some of those very same people were at the furniture sales yesterday." That caused us both to get a case of the giggles.

I was still holding the prescription in my hand when the medicine machine (I like to call it that) buzzed. "I'm done," I said proudly. As soon as the nurse came in and unhooked me, I tucked the prescription into my pocketbook. I would have done it earlier only I was afraid that I would pull the IV out of my hand. *Really brave, aren't I?* I thought to myself. *But thank God I have something that might help me, even if it helps just a little.*

"Onward and forward Rah," I jokingly said. Another doctor awaits my arrival. Oh lucky me." I got myself giggling because I was so relieved to get through another Chemo session. I know that the other patients receiving their treatments must have thought that I was nuts hearing me laugh so much, but I just couldn't help myself.

On the way to the car, and only after I had regained my composure, I asked Rah, "Do you suppose that one of the bags of medicine that is put in me through the IV is what this prescription is? Only now it is in pill form? I sure hope so, because I usually feel pretty good after the treatment, at least my stomach does."

"I don't know Mom, your guess is as good as anyone." Rah started up the car and we were on our way to doctor number two.

Chapter 38
A Good Day

As usual we reported on time at the radiation office. I saw Dr. Merrick as I was headed for my locker. He smiled and asked, "How are things going at chemotherapy?" I told him that things were going well and that I was having a good day so far." He smiled and walked into an exam room which held another unfortunate individual that was waiting for him. I wondered to my self, just how may poor people had gone through all this. Some of them recovering, and some just going through the motions, trying to hold on for that last chance of maybe they'll get better. "Stop it Pam, no need thinking like that." When your time comes, it comes. There is nothing that any human being can do to stop what the good Lord wants to happen.

Rah had gone to Susan's and hopefully will have something to eat. I was hopeful the appointments were on schedule as I wanted to escape as soon as possible. I hated Mondays. It was hard for everyone. Running here and there, keeping arrival times on schedule, having Dad watch the kids, all because I was sick. The whole thing was just a total disaster. *Damn cancer*, I thought, *your not going to get me. Not without one hell of a fight. Today I was in a fighting mode. I was feeling better as far as my stomach was concerned, which gave me my spunk back. I had been missing that a lot lately. I had just been to sick to care. But not today, today I was a walking talking fighting tiger!*

The radiation treatment went smoothly and quickly. I spoke with the same two nurses, (Teresa, and Mary) I finally asked them their names. I supposed if I were going to see them every day, and they knew my name I may as know them as well. We talked all during the treatment. I had to remember to lie perfectly still and, no arm movements. Now that is a very difficult little habit to change. I have always expressed my thoughts with my hands. Maybe it is from growing up in RI. We Rhode Islanders all seem to do it. But Teresa had threatened to tie my arms down, if I tried to move them, so I lay there, like a stiff board until the machine stopped.

Both of the ladies were very sweet, but I know that they were curious regarding my life. I gave them the short version, not wanting to share all the lousy details. I was divorced, had three children, seven grandchildren and one great-grandchild on the way. That rocked their socks. "How the heck old were you when you got married?" Mary asked.

"I had just turned eighteen, but I didn't have my first child until I was twenty."

Mary replied, "I should look so good when I become a grandmother."

"I look older than you and my daughter is only thirteen years old!"

I know that their questions, were just out of curiosity. They only wanted to get to know me a little better. They were two very kind and considerate women, and I was secretly hoping that we could become friends when all this nasty radiation business was completed.

On my return to change into my clothes, my thoughts were today had been a pretty good day. I had not had one of those types of days in a while. Now with the worry of the home behind me, my future didn't seem quite so dark. I can put all my concentration on getting well. No more extra added stress, just deal with the illness. I'm going to beat it. I know that I will. God is with me, as I can feel his presence with me every time I talk to him. I know that he is listening. He can hear my little voice and he gives me the strength to survive each day.

Just as I was leaving, I saw Dr. Merrick again. "Ms. Ayer, I want to see you tomorrow before you receive your treatment. Just dress as you normally do, only come in to this exam room before you report to the treatment room." he requested.

I immediately made an ugly face.

"What's the matter, don't want to see me?" he asked smiling.

"Oh it's not you, it's what you plan to do to me." I said teasingly.

He laughed right out loud. "See you tomorrow, Ms. Ayer."

"Bye Dr. Merrick, I said, and walked into the reception room.

I stepped outside, instead of Rah being there I saw Susan and the girls. "I almost did not recognize you at all. I was looking for Rah," I admitted.

Alex quickly commented, "Auntie Rah had to go home because Kyle (name) was sick and throwing up."

"Oh, poor Kyle (name) and poor Rah." was all I could muster.

We drove back to the house and Sue had prepared a very nice supper for us. Brandon had not come home as yet, but Sue was accustomed to his long hours. I just put his dinner in the oven, and he eats after he has been home for a while. I guess he just likes to unwind," Alex said acting like she was an adult.

"Pam, I didn't mean to pry but when I took the phone from the house you had a lot of messages on it. I only heard a couple of them before I shut it off, but one sounded important. It was someone from Providence Post Office, regarding your illness. They said that they needed additional information on the length of time you were going to be out. I wrote the number down for you. I am sorry, but I think that it was a lucky thing that I heard the message, or it might have been erased when I unplugged the phone. I hope you're not upset with me, because I really didn't mean to do it.," she confessed.

"Oh Sue, don't be ridiculous." I wanted to check the messages myself, but I didn't have the courage. I will call the number tomorrow and provide the phone number here so they may reach me if any questions arise. I am sure that if they need any medical information, I can get it tomorrow from Dr. Merrick." I knew that Sue was felt upset about listening to my messages, but it didn't bother me one bit, and I tried to get that message across to her. She was a very sensitive girl, and she was frightened I would be angry. *Silly girl*, I thought. *She doesn't really know me yet, but she will.*

I told Sue and the girls that I was going to go to my room for a while. I was actually feeling pretty good, but I was tired. "Sue, I have a prescription that has to be filled, and I hate to ask you but I really need it. Supposedly it is going to stop my vomiting and my diarrhea."

Sue quickly said, "No problem Pam, the girls and I will go right now."

"You don't have to go right this minute," I added.

"What drug store do you use Pam?" Sue asked.

"Bricks Drug store in Johnston," I replied.

"We have one of those right down the road. You go rest a while, and by the time you feel better, we'll be back with your medicine. Do you have your medical card handy?" she asked.

"Yes, it's right in my purse. Hold on a second and I will get it for you."

Bri spoke, "I'll get your pocketbook Meme. Is it in your bedroom?"

Yes it is little one, thank you," I said smiling at her. I couldn't help but think how very sweet these little girls are. Always trying to please. That is very rare these days. "Sue, you don't have to take the girls, unless they want to go. They can stay here with me," I confessed.

"No, you go get some rest, besides they love to shop. They take after me, at least that is what your son would say," Sue admitted teasingly. Both of the girls readily admitted they wanted to stay home with me. So, Sue was off all by her self and the girls and I went downstairs to watch some tv and talk. We had always had our special time together; just me and all of the female grandchildren. They would stay over to my house and we would talk about everything. We would stay up late, cook marshmallows and they would tell on their mothers and fathers. I would usually end up laughing until I had tears in my eyes as a result of the stories the girls told me. Tawnee and Alex were the same age, and Bri and Haley were only one year apart. So they would kind of pair off and the older two would go in one room and play, while the younger two girls would be playing something totally different. We really had a lot of fun, and I had such a special bond with all of them. They are so very special to me, each and every one.

Alex was lying next to me on my bed and Bri was sitting at my vanity testing all my perfumes. She took my hair brush and began to brush her hair. Both Alex and Bri had gorgeous hair. Susan had seen to it that their hair had never been cut since they were babies. Both of these little girls had been taught how to take care of their own hair. They washed their hair every night and spent at least an hour drying and brushing it. Sue had instructed them well how to be little ladies, and the importance of hygiene. It was also decided there would be no hair cuts (only the ends trimmed) until they reached the age of eighteen. Both Alex and Bri never went anywhere until they were "dressed to the nines" and their hair perfectly styled. It was really amazing to see the reactions of strangers when they looked at them. People always commented on how beautiful they were. Brandon and Sue were so proud of them, but boy were they going to be in for trouble when these little girls grew up. I pray every night, that I will be able to see all of my granddaughters as adult, mature women.

About fifteen minutes had elapsed when the noise of a loud truck pulling into the driveway occurred. I went to the window but could not see what name was written on the delivery truck. The girls and I scurried to the front door and a man stepped out of the truck and came to the door with a clipboard. When I opened the door, he inquired if this was the Ayer residence?

"Yes, it is," I admitted.

"I have a delivery for you, where do you want it?"

"What is it?" I asked. But before he could answer Susan drove in and jumped out of her car and yelled to the man. He walked over to her, leaving me standing there in the door way. After a brief conversation with Sue, he turned and walked toward the back of the truck. I could hear the rear door of his truck being opened.

Sue walked over to me and said, "Oh, it's something for Brandon's work." I didn't give the subject another thought. We just turned around and proceeded to climb the stairs. Another ten minutes or so elapsed, when I heard the door of the truck slam and the beeping sound of a truck backing out of the drive away.

Sue was standing at the window and said "Pam, you should see what that driver left in our driveway."

"What did he leave? What is it?" I asked as I walked over to the window.

Alex and Bri started jumping and yelling "Surprise, Meme!"

I looked out the window and what I saw was the last thing I would have ever expected to see. What was stacked in the driveway, was an entire bathroom. There was a toilet, an enclosed shower stall, a sink and mirrored cabinet. "Oh my God!" was all I could say.

"Surprise, surprise, surprise!" was echoed through the house.

We walked down the stairs and went outside. I was crying uncontrollably. I realize that most women wouldn't cry over a toilet, but it was as beautiful to me as a diamond ring would have been to another woman. Both Alex and Bri were hugging me and trying to console me.

"It's alright. I am crying because I am so happy." I explained to them.

Bri was so filled with excitement she blurted out, "There is another surprise too!"'

"Another surprise, I don't think I can take another one."

Right then Brandon drove in and he was driving my car. My Eagle Talon, the car I loved so much. "Oh, my car," I yelled. I was yelling louder than the girls. "My car is here, I have my car back." Suddenly reality hit me, I saw the look on Brandon's face. He was not smiling, not smiling at all.

Brandon got out of the car and walked over to me. "Mom, I am so sorry, but the car company called and they are coming to repossess your car tomorrow. The only way they won't take it is if you pay them $900 in cash tomorrow when they arrive. You can use your furniture money if you choose, it's your money, your decision."

I know that my expression must have changed instantly, as the girls were once again by my side. "Please don't cry Meme," Alex asked.

Bri was quick to add, "Meme, that's not the second surprise I told you about."

Sue snapped at the girls and told them "go into the house right now." Both the girls moved immediately. When their mother uses that tone, there is no arguing allowed.

Brandon said, "Please Mom, we should go in the house and sit down and talk for a minute."

I looked at him sadly and said, "Brandon, let them take it. We need the money for the apartment. "There is no other choice that one. I need a home much more than I need that car. It's only a car. Someday I'll replace it...perhaps in another time or in another life." I put my head on my sons shoulder and cried my heart out. *So much for a good day*, I thought to myself, *but I have a beautiful bathroom in the driveway!*

Chapter 39
My Wonderful
Brother...Edward

We all sat outside and talked for a while longer, but the temperature started to drop, and we decided to go inside. Besides, Brandon had all that bathroom equipment to moved inside the house. "Your not going to move that alone are you?" I asked him.

"No, my friends Joe and Peter should be here any minute to help me with it. "Mom, you and Sue go inside, I will wait out here for my friends to arrive" "They should be here any minute." Within ten minutes both of the boys arrived. All three of them began to carry in all the equipment that was destined to be my new bathroom. I was on the living room couch, surrounded by my little grandchildren who were very concerned about my tears.

"Are you okay, Meme?" Alex asked.

I looked at her and she had tears in her eyes. "Now I don't want to see you cry." I scolded her. "That makes me feel worse, so look at me and give me a smile."

"It's only a silly old car. Nothing is more important than my family and for me to get well," I said giving her a squeeze.

Bri quietly said, "If I were rich, I would buy you a car Meme."

"Thank you little one, I know you would. But promise me we shall not worry about that old car anymore. I am going to have my very own bathroom downstairs, hurray" I said smiling. "Your daddy is going to make it beautiful for me."

"Yes, he will, Alex agreed smiling.

Brandon and his friends were finished within minutes of their arrival. Up the stairs they all came, and they sounded like a herd of elephants. Had it been the girls that made that much noise, they would have most certainly been scolded. But boys will be boys, even if they are grown men. Brandon's friend Joe saw me sitting on the couch, and said "Hello Mrs. Ayer, you look wonderful as usual."

"Thank you Joe," I said. But I thought to myself, he is so full of bull. He always was ever since he was a small boy. He and Brandon had been friends since early childhood. He idolized Brandon, and on occasion Brandon had to avoid him like the plague because Joe didn't know when to go home.

Brandon entered the room, and in his usual commanding voice stated, "Mom, I am planning to start working on your bathroom Thursday. My boss advised me today that I could have Thursday through Monday off. I should be able to have your bathroom up and operational by Saturday, if I don't run encounter any major problems.

"That was very nice of your boss Brandon, but can you afford to be absent from work?"

"I'm getting paid for it Mom, so don't get nervous," he said proudly.

"Well, I don't want you to overextend yourself either," I said fulling utilizing my mothers authoritative voice. Brandon just smiled.

His friends offered their goodbyes to all, and promised their return on Friday afternoon to assist Brandon with the bathroom. I sat there and wondered if Brandon's friends and his boss knew about my illness. I would put money on it, but Brandon is funny sometimes. I don't think he would tell anyone about his personal problems, but it might have been Sue. Sue has no trouble in speaking her mind, and probably never will. Sue states exactly what she thinks; whether or not you want to hear it.

Brandon turned to me after his friends left and said, "Mom, about the car."

My immediate reply was, "I told you how I wanted it handled. Let's just drop it."

"But I want to explain something to you."Brandon interrupted. "The only reason that I brought your car to this house was because the repossession company's office is in Fairfield. If they had to send a truck out to Clayson to pick it up, they would charge you a lot of money. This was the only way that you won't be charged. Besides, I didn't want them to take it away without giving you the chance to keep it, if that is what you wanted to do."

"I understand Brandon," I said, Don't worry about it. I only want to make sure that I am not here when they come to pick it up. I don't want to see it happen," I admitted.

Sue spoke said, "I'll take you anywhere you want to go tomorrow after your radiation treatments. I will make sure that you will not have to witness your car being removed."

Bri asked her father, "Can I tell Meme now, about her surprise?"

Brandon smiled and said, "Yes, go ahead before you burst."

"I forgot you told me there was another surprise, Bri." I said smiling. Please tell me quickly, I want to here all about it."

Sue spoke before Bri could, "Your brother Ed, paid for your bathroom. Apparently he called your mother, or she could have called him, but the point is he has full knowledge of your illness. He phoned here and I spoke with him. He obviously hung up after speaking with me, contacted the supplier, and purchased everything over the phone. " But that is not the surprise," Sue said. Go ahead Alex and Bri, tell her what the surprise is."

"Your brother is going to be here to see you on Friday." they yelled. "Surprise.!!!"

"My brother is coming here to see me? I exclaimed. I haven't seen him in about over five years!" Brandon went on to explain, "He phoned and we spoke Saturday night. He was very worried about your illness, and was crying on the phone. He really loves you very much, Mom," Brandon added.

"He does? He really does?" I asked.

"Yes, Mom, he really does. Why shouldn't he," Sue asked.

I know that might have sounded stupid to Brandon and Sue, but I had always loved my brother so very much. He left home when I was very young, and Edward was only seventeen himself at that time. He lived a life that I could only dream about. I had secretly wished that I was just like him. He was always carefree and happy. He went anywhere he wanted and I was sure that he did not suffer from panic attacks. He had married a wonderful woman, and now that they both had retired, and they were traveling the world.

I missed him so much sometimes. Sure we teased each other, and he used to tell me that I was adopted. But that was just Edward. He was tall, fair skinned and light eyes, and I was almost the total opposite. He had lost his hair and the early age of twenty. The baldness trait was from my real fathers side of the family and Edward inherited that gene. If I should lose my hair, he would have his total revenge on me, because that was the only weapon I could use against him, I had hair. I smiled just thinking how he would take advantage of the fact that I was now bald like him. Of course it would all be in jest, but he would not let the opportunity pass him by, of that I was totally convinced.

The only thing we really had in common was our sense of humor. We could drive our mother crazy with it. As I stated earlier, poor Mom did not have much of a sense of humor. She would threaten us with everything she could think of to make us stop teasing her, but we would be relentless.

I was so excited at just the thought of him coming to Rhode Island to see me. I finally know that he really does love me and does worry about me. It wasn't exactly the way I wanted to determine that fact, but I would take it.

I asked Brandon, "Do you know if Fern (Edwards wife) is coming with him?"

"No, he didn't say. That will have to be another surprise," Brandon said smiling.

I had always loved and admired Fern. She and Edward met when he was working in Canada. She is a beautiful girl, a talented artist and a registered nurse. How she tolerated with my brother all those years, or even why she would find him attractive was beyond anyone's guess.

"I wonder where they are going to stay," Sue asked. They can stay here if they don't mind sleeping on the couch," Brandon said.

"Oh no, I have a better idea, I can sleep with the girls and they can sleep in my bedroom." I stated. "Well, we won't worry about that until they get here. The important thing is that they are coming, so smile Mom."

My immediate response was, "I will Brandon. This news helps me a lot right now, and I can use all the help available."

I decided to change the subject right as my pain suddenly reminded me it was time for a pill.

"Sue did you get my prescription for me?"

"Oh yes, I totally forgot about them when I pulled in the driveway and saw the delivery truck." She reached for her purse and pulled out my new pills and returned my medical card. "Better put this away, so you don't lose it, Pam," Sue instructed.

"I will, don't be such a worry wart." I said laughing. The new prescription was named something I couldn't even attempt to pronounce. I thought, I will research this on our next visit to the library with Sue and the kids. That reminded me to ask Sue, "Can you take me to the library one day this week? I really need to find out some information regarding cervical cancer. Of course, we usually go on Thursday afternoon. Is Thursday alright?" Sue asked.

"Thursday is fine." I was glad that I had finally remembered to set up a time to visit the library. My questions regarding where and how I got my cancer was eating away at me, and I didn't want to ask the doctors. I wanted to read all I could about the cancer first, so when they began explaining it to me, I would be able to accept their explanations.

"Sue, I might be longer than usual tomorrow at the doctors." Dr. Merrick told me today that he wants to examine me before my treatment. So I am not sure how long I will be there."

Her reply was, "Don't worry about it, I will drop you off and you can call me when you are ready to come home. I'm only around the corner, remember?"

I was really dreading the exam tomorrow. I was afraid of what I was going to hear, and the pain was unbearable. I actually began having nightmares about the exams and the pain. But I can take it, I thought. I am Pam, and I am strong. My constant prayer was, please God, give me strength.

Brandon suddenly asked, "Is anybody hungry but me?"

Alex and Bri both yelled " I am."

"Alex suggested her favorite, "Let's have pizza?"

Brandon looked at me and I smiled, "Pizza it is."

"Let's go girls. Well be back in a flash with the pizza."

After they had left Sue asked me, "Pam are you going to eat pizza?"

"No, as much as I love it, I don't dare."

"Well how about if I make you a bowl of soup?" she asked.

"Sue, that would be wonderful." I said with a smile.

Brandon and the girls were only gone for a short time. The Pizza Palace was only a short distance from their home, but I had already finished my soup. When they came up the stairs carrying the boxes of pizza, (yes, two boxes) the smell was wonderful. How I would have loved to eat about two good sized pieces, but not yet, I thought. Just as soon as I get better, I shall eat until I pop.

"I'm going downstairs now, I am really tired from all the excitement. Everyone have a good night and I will see you all in the morning. And yes, I will call you if I need anything at all," I said smiling at both Brandon and Sue. I walked down the stairs and into the unfinished part of the basement. I could see my big screen tv sitting over in the left corner of the room, and right beside it was my refrigerator. Both of them Brandon had covered with my old bedspread. *Brandon thinks of everything*, I thought. *He must have inherited all his brains from me. That thought made me smile. Sure Pam, take all the credit, you did all the work. You carried him, you raised him and you loved him. No wonder he became the man he is.*

I walked over to all my new bathroom equipment. I ran my hand over the porcelain toilet. "You beautiful little white life saver," I said out loud. "I shall hug my brother as I have never hugged him before, and I shall tell him how much I love him as I always have." I hadn't realized how much I had missed him all these years. Yes, he was always in my thoughts, but I never thought about a day when I might not be able to see him ever again. I know that he would have been devastated if we had not been able to say goodby. So no matter what happens from here on, I will have had to the chance to tell my brother how much he means to me. And that is a good thing.

I walked to my bedroom window and looked at my car. I smiled because I had some special memories concerning it. I used to put all my grandchildren in it, we would slide the top open, roll down all the windows, and I would put in a tape of some old fashioned good ole rock and roll songs from the 50's. The kids would sing at the top of their voices and bob their little heads up and down to the music. Oh how we would laugh. They would yell, louder Meme, louder. That is how I will remember my Eagle Talon. Singing with my grandchildren.

But in remembering the Talon I also thought of a question for Brandon. I moved slowly to the bottom of the staircase and yelled, "Brandon, can you clean my car out before the repossession man gets here? I have some of my favorite tapes in it and probably a lot of other things I just can't remember right now?" Brandon yelled down his answer," Already have everything in a box Mom. I just have to bring it inside tonight. I've got it covered. Stop worrying and go to bed," he commanded.

"Yes sir," I answered. I returned to my bedroom and did exactly what I was told. I thought, *what a good girl I am. I still take orders no matter who is giving them.* I fell asleep picturing the kids singing the rock and rolls songs.

Chapter 40

Pretty Underwear vs Boxer Shorts

I was up and at the kitchen table by 6:30 a.m. My usual attire was my bathrobe with my urgently required morning coffee. Brandon was the first one out of his bedroom, "I thought I smelled coffee," he said with a grumpy tone. "What are you doing up so early Mother?"

I just couldn't sleep," I answered.

His voice sounded concerned now, "Are you feeling alright?'

I thought about telling a small lie, but then admitted, "Not really. I am feeling extremely weak, but not sick to my stomach."

Sue walked into the kitchen and joined the conversation. "Not doing to well this morning Pam?"

"No, I was just admitting that to Brandon, I feel extremely weak and light headed."

Sue asked, "Did you have anything to eat besides the coffee that you have sitting in front of you, which I might add you shouldn't be drinking?"

I couldn't seem to hold my head up any longer, so I just laid it down on the table. "I'll be alright, I think this feeling will pass if I just give it a little time," I said hopefully.

"Can I do anything for you? Perhaps some crackers or something along that line of food. You really should eat something." Sue said.

My voice began to crack, "I just don't think I can handle this. I am trying to be strong, but this illness is getting to me."

Sue asked, "Where has the "I won't give up," and" I can do this," attitude gone?" "Is the stubbornness and determination gone as well?"

"I am just so very physically weak this morning, I confessed. Please don't make me go this morning for my treatment. Can't I just skip today, just today?" I asked pitifully.

Brandon was angry and scared, he said, "Not on your life, you are not skipping a treatment even if I have to call an ambulance to get you there."

"Okay, okay, I am not going to argue, just let me keep my head down for a few more minutes," I pleaded. Brandon stormed out and returned to his bedroom. "I have upset him Sue, and I am so sorry," I said crying.

Sue sat down beside me and held my hand, "It's not Brandon that you have to worry about, please, just this once, care about yourself." Sue pleaded.

"Alright, if you can help me get into the bathroom, I think a shower might help me." I asked. I tried to stand up but the room began spinning and my knees buckled. I went right down to the floor and landed on my rear end.

Sue yelled," Brandon, get in here. Your mother needs you now!" His face was reflecting total fear when he saw me on the floor.

"Oh my God, Sue call the ambulance," he shouted.

"No, I forbid it. I will be alright if I can just get into the bathroom," I said. Brandon came over to me, his hands were shaking. He reached down and put his arms under my arms and gently pulled me to my feet. "Just help me to get in the bathroom," I pleaded.

"Okay Mom, whatever you want." Brandon said softly. We walked very slowly to the bathroom door. I held on to the door, and told Brandon, " I could make it from there." He looked hesitant, but did as I requested. I took a few steps and then closed the door. I held on to the sink and made my way to the toilet seat and sat down. "I'm alright and I am sitting down." I yelled. If I need your help, I promise that I will yell out for you. I think I am feeling a little better," I lied.

I could hear their voices in the kitchen. I thought, *well you really did it this morning Pam. Nice job of hiding your sickness from your son. I should get a handle on this acting healthy or they will send me to the hospital and that is the last place I want to be. I sat there on the toilet seat for a short period of time, and then reached into the tub to turn on the water to begin my shower. I know the shower would help me, it always has. But recently all these new side effects are happening, and I never know what to expect. How can I hide something, when I don't know it's coming or even what new symptoms are going to appear? I did my usual crying sitting on the floor of the tub. It was at that moment that I noticed hair rushing into the drain. Oh no,* I thought. It has finally started to happen. I placed my hands on top of my head and gently began fluffing my hair. I brought my hands back to the front of my face, expecting to see huge globs of brown hair stuck between my finger tips. But there was nothing there but shampoo suds. What is going on? I looked toward the drain and again I saw more hair. I slowly pulled myself to an upright position, still looking down. It was at that moment I saw the source of the hair! Let me just say this, it was in a totally different area than my head. I can handle that, I thought. At least I won't have to worry about wearing a bathing suit and a bikini wax. I began to laugh, half crying and half laughing.

Sue came to the door and asked, "are you okay in there?"

"Better," I said. "I'll explain when I am finished with my shower." I slowly began to feel better. At least the weakness was fading. I walked into the kitchen with a towel wrapped around my head and my ugly bathrobe on.

"Mom, you scared me to death," Brandon admitted.

"I'm sorry, I didn't mean to scare the both of you, but I think that the treatments are beginning to take an effect on my body as well as the tumor."

"It's to be expected, and we have to get used to it. I wish you didn't have to witness my pain, I just couldn't hide it this morning. Right now I am still a little wobbly, so if one of you could just guide me downstairs, I shall get dressed," I said reassuring them with my I'm okay smile. Sue jumped up and assisted me in going to my bedroom. "Help me to be strong Sue, just like you did this morning. Yell at me, and don't let me get the "I give up attitude," not even for a few minutes." I pleaded.

Sue's curiosity had finally reached it's peak, "What were you laughing at when you were in the bathroom? First I heard crying and then laughter. Are you losing it Pam?" she asked smiling.

"No, I am not losing it. After I get dressed, I will explain it to you, I said smirking. Your going to get a huge kick out of my answer."

The phone was ringing as I walked into my bedroom, and it was my son Jay. "Just checking in on you Mom, how are you doing?"

"Doing fine, so far so good, I lied. I do know for sure the treatments are going to be a long drawn out experience.

"Did the doctor tell you that?" Jay asked.

"Not in so many words, however my conversations with the nurses and other patients it appears that cancer takes time to kill I confessed. Not to worry though, you know how tough I am. How's that beautiful little Cheyenne doing?" I asked.

"She's fine and so is Ann. We were just concerned about you. Please call me and let me know what is going on," he requested.

"Did you know that my brother is coming to see me," I said excitedly?

"Yes, I know all about it. Nana gave me all the information regarding Uncle Edwards arrival."

"I want you and Ann to come and visit when he gets here." I told him." I stated emphatically.

"Oh we will Mom, don't worry about that. It's been a long time since I have seen him too," he admitted.

"Jay, I have to get ready for my doctors appointment, but I will call you as soon as Edward arrives, okay?"

"Alright Mom, I will talk to you later, bye and love you."

"Bye son, I love you too." I had to move quickly after the phone conversation as my time was limited this morning. Even with getting my early start, my crying spells had slowed me down considerably. I moved as rapidly as my body would allow. My hair and my make-up were done, and I looked at myself in the mirror once again. I still look like a scarecrow no matter how hard I try, I admitted to myself. But the weight will return once this new medicine gets into my system. If I can just stop vomiting and going to the bathroom all the time, the weight will reappear on my bones. I left my bedroom with a much better attitude and started walking towards the stairway. Sue and the girls were on their way down the stairs by the time I reached the door way. Sue immediately said, "Pam you look much better than you did. Are you feeling stronger now, or is it just the make-up?"

I confessed, "It's mostly the make-up, but mentally I do feel better now."

"Okay, tell me now why your were laughing in the bathroom,"" Sue asked.

"Sue, let me put it to you this way. I do not have to get a bikini wax this summer, as the Chemo has taken care of that type of bathing suit precaution." She looked at me strangely at first, and then it registered what I was saying. I did not want to say it outright in front of the girls.

"Oh no, not down there?" she asked.

"Better there than on my head," I said laughing. As we approached the car, Sue and I were still laughing and smiling. The girls were totally lost by our private joke, but they joined in our laughter anyway.

The children were so good for me, both physically and mentally. Their effect on me was nothing but positive. They showed me every minute they were with me, how much they loved me. How could anyone ask for more than that to survive the day?

We arrived at the radiation building on time, and kissed the girls and hugged Sue. "I'll call you when I am finished. I might be a while, as I have to see the dreaded doctor," I said jokingly.

"Alright, I will await your call," Sue replied. They were already departing by the time I reached the front door of the building.

I walked immediately to the locker room and changed into my radiation outfit (I like to refer to it as that). I approached the first nurse that I saw in the hallway. "Do you know where Dr. Merrick is this morning?"I asked

"I believe that he is in the second exam room on the left."

"Thank you," and I continued on my journey to the dreaded examination table. I strolled into the exam room and Dr Merrick was no where to be seen. I thought well, I may as well get myself on the table. There is no way of escaping the inevitable! As I sat there, my heart was racing and my knees were knocking. I hope I don't have to sit here too long, as I don't think I can stand waiting. My wish was granted and into the room Dr. Merrick appeared. "Good morning, Ms. Ayer." he said in his usual good natured tone of oice. "Feeling a little edgy this morning?" he asked. How can he tell that I wondered to myself? "Your knees are very visibly knocking," he teased.

"It shows that much? I thought that I was doing a wonderful job hiding the fact that I am scared to death. I was positive that I had the knees under control," I confessed.

"Well, try and make sure that your knees don't crash into the side of my head, while I am examining you, okay?" he requested jokingly. I couldn't control my laughter even with how nervous I was. I burst into laughter and so did he.

"Now, just relax and I will be as quick and painless as I can possibly be." he stated.

"Alright doctor, I shall give it my best." He did not exaggerate at all. The exam was completed in record time, without any serious amount of discomfort. He removed his rubber gloves and the magnifying glasses and washed his hands, never saying a word. My heart was pounding. "What's the matter?" I asked. "Is the tumor worse?"

He smiled and simply said, "On the contrary, there has been significant visible improvement in the tumor. I am very pleased, as well you should be too."

"Oh thank God, doctor." I said smiling.

"We shall continue to proceed as we have been doing. Any questions, or problems?" he asked.

"Only one," I answered. As you have already seen, I have lost all the hair in that area, but I am very uncomfortable down there. "Is there any medication or cream I can use, as I am getting severely burned," I confessed being very embarrassed.

"I can help you with that problem. I will write you out a prescription which you can pick it up at the receptionist desk when you leave today."

"Thank you very much doctor."

Dr Merrick then offered me some advise, "You might want to change your underwear from what you are wearing. No more pretty sexy underpanties, try boxer shorts. They will be much more comfortable and assist your problem and eliminate your discomfort."

"What? Give up my sexy underwear? It's all I have left to feel pretty?" I said panic stricken.

"Yes, it is for your own comfort." he stated firmly. You shall have plenty of time to feel sexy and pretty when you fully regain your health." he admitted.

"Hmp!" was my disappointed reaction. "Boxer shorts? Are you sure you mean "Boxer shorts? Oh that is going to be attractive," I added.

He smiled at me and simply said, "They will be much more comfortable during your future treatments."

He changed the subject and asked me about my pain? "Has the pain lessened?"

"Well, I am really not sure," I confessed. I take my pills right on schedule, which is every four hours."

"Let me suggest an alternative. Take your medication only when you need it, and determine the level of your pain without a pain pill. Please, record the schedules in order for us to determine when the level of pain and how much it decreases."

I agreed to follow his instructions, and then I asked, "Is that it for today?"

"Yes, I think that is it," he was smiling, and he opened the door and left the room.

I left the exam room and went immediately to the location of the radiation treatment center. I saw my two familiar nurses, Teresa and Mary standing and talking. "I am sorry that I am a little late, but I had to see Dr. Merrick." Mary smiled and said, "Don't worry about that. We knew where you were."

I told them of the doctors instructions. Teresa began to laugh, but then she caught herself, and tried to contain her humor. "He would never give you bad advise, and I am sure he is correct in prescribing boxer shorts. The three of us started laughing quiet loudly. Dr. Merrick leaned out of the doorway where was standing and just gave us all a huge grin. He knew exactly what we were discussing. "I will show him some boxer shorts, I said devilishly. Just wait until tomorrow."

The treatment went very well, and I was off the table in a very few minutes. I shared my news recounting Dr. Merrick's statements regarding my tumor. Teresa said, "That's wonderful news, Pam."

"Yes it is, isn't it? I admitted. I can hardly wait until I get home and call everyone with the good news. Mary commented, "Pam, remember you still have a long way to go, but any improvement is worthy of a celebration, so go ahead and celebrate."

"Thank you, both. I intend to thank the good Lord with a special conversation tonight. I have already thanked him numerous times today, but one more thank you can't hurt." With that on my mind, I returned to the locker room to change clothes and to start calling the family. But first I have to make a stops, before I let Sue bring me home. I can't wait to tell everyone, and I smiled as I walked out of the building and headed for Sue's car.

How did it go today?" Sue asked as I climbed in the car.

"Oh Sue, the doctor said my tumor is reacting very quickly to the treatments," I said excitedly.

"Thank God, Pam," Sue said as she started to cry.

"I already have, thanked him Sue. Believe me. I already have. But, and there always a but, it is still very early in the treatment and I have a long way to go." I admitted. It has certainly turned out to be a wonderful day. I said happily. Sue, can we make a couple to stops before we go home? I have another prescription that has to be filled, plus I need to go to the Mall to buy something."

Sue gave me a funny look, "the Mall? Are you up to the Mall?" she asked.

"I just have to go in one store and purchase something, it will only take a minute," please I asked? "Okay, as long as you are strong enough."she agreed and started the car.

Sue left the prescription at the pharmacy and informed the pharmacist that she would pick it up later in the day. The Mall was a short drive from the radiation building and the drug store. "Which store do you want to visit Pam?" Sue asked.

"It really doesn't matter, any one of the big department stores," I said eagerly. Pick ever which one where we may park close to the building."

Sue just looked at me funny again and said, "Okay."

Once we were in the Mall, I knew exactly where I was going. I explained to Sue while we were walking, that I was in search of boxer shorts. I provided all the details of my conversation with Dr. Merrick regarding my underwear. Sue had all she could do not to laugh out loud. "Well, I am going to find some boxer shorts that will cause him some laughter," I told her. I narrowed my search to the boys underwear department . Low and behold, I saw a large assortment of them hanging up against the wall. I never dreamed that there was such a large assortment of cartoon character boxer shorts. I picked out five different styles with an assortment of cartoons imprinted upon them. My favorite one (which I decided I had to have two of) was the "Smiley Face." Needless to say, the shopping spree caused a generous amount of giggles between myself and Sue.

We returned to the drug store in record time and Sue went inside to retrieve my prescription. As I sat in the car waiting, I kept thinking, I must find out about my car, and when Sue returned to the car

I asked, "Did the repossession company come and take my car?" The look on her face, gave me the answer. "Never mind, I already know just by looking at you."

"I'll think about that tomorrow...."

Chapter 41
My Brother Arrives

Upon our arrival at home, I remembered that I had to return the call from the Post Office, I had forgotten all about it. I asked Sue, "Do you still have the phone number that was left on the answering machine?"

"Yes, I do, I wrote down in my notebook which I keep in my purse, " she quickly replied. "I'll get it for you right now."

I was fairly confident that I knew what the post office wanted, but as with everything else in life, you never know for sure. Sue returned to the kitchen with the phone number. "Here goes," I said wearily. "Personnel Department, this is Marie, how may I help you?"

"Hi Marie, this is Pam Ayer."

"I received your message that you called."

"Oh, yes Pam."

"How are you?" she said in a concerned tone of voice.

"I am okay, what is that you need from me?"

"We need another form completed by your doctor regarding the extent and length of your illness," she replied.

"I can give you his name and address right now, and you can mail the form directly to him."

"That would be great," she said being very agreeable.

I gave her Dr. Merrick's name and address, along with his phone number. "If you need any further information, I am staying at my son's home and I will give you the phone number here."

"Please don't hesitate to call me with any other questions you might incur in the future." I gave her Brandon's number and said goodbye. "That's a good job done, I thought. Let Dr. Merrick's secretary do all the formal paperwork for which the post office was famous for.

After hanging up the phone, I looked at Sue and replied, "Sue, I have to fill out a change of address form" How stupid is that?" Here I am a Postmaster and I didn't think to handle such an important thing. Sue was very calm and simply said, "I think you have had other things on your mind recently. I can handle it for you later on today. Don't give in another thought."

The phone rang and it was my mother. "Hi Mom," I said with my ususal happy voice. "How are things going?" she asked before I could say another word. I advised her of all the latest developments regarding my tumor. "When did you find all this out?" she asked.

"Just a short while ago, I just came in the door. I was going to call everyone and give the good news to all of you."

"Do you want me to call Rah and tell her?" she said hopefully.

"You can if you choose, I will call Jay, and then I am going to lie down for a while. I am feeling very tired," I confessed.

"Alright then, you call Jay and I'll call Rah," she said confirming her job.

"I call you later this evening Mom, after I take a nap."

I planned on retiring early this evening. Even with the nap, sleeping all night had been coming to me easier because of the medication. I had started the regime of monitoring my pain pills as Dr. Merrick had suggested. I had taken one this afternoon and felt the need to take one now. It is 10 o'clock. There has been a little improvement, I thought to myself. Today I had only taken three pills, and that is a decisively decreased amount. Normally, I would just take them every four hours as prescribed. I was beginning to feel that Dr. Merrick was absolutely correct.

I placed my clothes for the morning carefully on the chair next to my vanity. My new Boxer shorts were in my underwear drawer awaiting to be worn. I was going to wait for the right day to wear them. My plan was to wait until I was to see Dr. Merrick again for another exam, but I was beginning to feel very uncomfortable in my lower region. I may be required to put my pretty underwear away faster than I originally planned. I shut my light off, and began a long conversation with the Lord. There was so much that I had to thank him for tonight. My vomiting had ceased, and my diarrhea had also improved. My tumor was beginning to shrink, and I had the beginning of a home. Best of all, my brother was coming to see me. So much to be thankful for. I must of fallen asleep while talking to God, as the next thing I remembered was my alarm clock buzzing.

Today was Friday, and I was finally going to see my brother. I was so excited that nothing else mattered to me. My pain or my discomfort was not going to sway my happiness. But I knew that I had to keep myself calm and my emotions in check. First things first. I must get through the treatment this morning. My weakness had returned, and I was feeling much the same as yesterday morning. Today would have been the day that I go to Rah's house, but she and Sue had determined that it would be better with Edward's visit, that I remain until Sunday night. Rah must have called Sue, while I was taking a nap late yesterday afternoon. Sue had come down stairs and asked me if I thought it was a good idea to follow that plan. I agreed, as Sue and Brandon's house was far more suitable for company. Rah did not have any room for Edward and Fern to sleep and I didn't know if Fern was accompanying Edward on this trip.

Very carefully I made my journey upstairs. I held the railing very tightly to keep my balance. Sue was already up, and had made the coffee. "Your coffee is ready and waiting for you Pam, but I really wish you would try and eat something this morning," she asked.

"I was just thinking the same thing. I would like to try and eat a good breakfast if you wouldn't mind making it for me?"

"Great, she said. I'll start with some scrambled eggs and bacon for you right now."

"Let me just drink my coffee and then get into the shower, I suggested. I always feel better after I have showered."

Sue smiled and said, "take your time."

While I was sipping my coffee, Brandon came into the kitchen. He was already dressed and looked prepared to go to work. "Mom, I want you to stay up here today as much as possible."

"I am going to start working on the bathroom this morning."

"I will be doing a lot of dry wall work, and that creates a lot of dust particles flying around." I don't think that it is a good idea for you to be breathing in all that junk in your weakened condition," he said acting very concerned and determined. I would like to think that I can accomplish this while you are at your treatment this morning. So no argument from you is allowed. If Edward arrives, you can enjoy your visit right up here. There is no reason for you to be in the basement. Also, tonight you can sleep with the girls, and not downstairs. How do you like that for orders?"

"I agree with you, I said smiling. Fooled you didn't I? You think I don't know what you are really thinking. You just want me totally out of your way, so that I can't drive you crazy when your working. I know you Sonny boy, I said. But I agree with you and I will not go down stairs until you tell me that it is okay. Besides, when Edward arrives he will probably want to go visit Mom and Dad and everyone else. So we will be out of your hair, at least for a while. Agreed?" I asked.

"Yes, sounds good," Brandon replied.

Sue asked, "Don't you think Edward will want to see the bathroom equipment that he purchased?" Brandon smiled, "He is allowed down there, not Mom."

My shower felt very soothly this morning. I was extremely excited about seeing my brother. I smiled as the water fell all over my body. This is an usual moment, I thought. Most of the time that I spend in the shower, I am crying. I shall cherish this moment and store it in my memory for the future mornings to come.

My pain was at an acceptable level this morning . I shall wait until after breakfast before I considered taking any medication. If my body pain was tolerable, the pill would have to wait. Alex and Bri were seated at the kitchen table wearing their beautiful smiles and lovely school clothes. "Hi Meme," they echoed.

"Good morning my little pumpkins," I replied smiling. Are you ready to meet your Uncle Edward?" Bri spoke up, "Yep, Mommy tells me he is funny."

"Yes, that he is little one. You will like him, but be careful he usually has some tricks up his sleeves."

"What kind of tricks?" Alex asked.

"You just never know, but don't say I didn't warn you," I said laughing. We finished breakfast, which was excellent. Sue is a very good cook, but I had some difficulty in finishing every thing on my plate. But I thought that I did fairly well when you consider my sensitive stomach.

I kissed the girls good bye and Sue and I started for the stairs to leave for my treatment. I could already hear Brandon working. The sound of the saw was already audible.

"I am glad that I won't be downstairs today."

"That sound would drive my crazy and give me a major head ache."

Sue just smiled and said, "lucky me."

The treatment was quick and painless this morning. I shared my excitement with Teresa and Mary regarding the arrival of my brother. I think that I did a lot of babbling as I could not contain my enthusiasm. Both the ladies just smiled and wished that I should have a great time visiting with my brother and fully enjoy my weekend. I did my usual changing of clothes and then left the building. Sue was awaiting me in the parking lot.

Once I got into the car, the first question I asked her was, "have you heard anything from Edward?" "Nothing yet Pam, but I am sure that he is on his way," she said trying her best to reassure me. "Besides, it's still very early in the morning, and he probably won't arrive until later this afternoon."

"Try and relax and stay calm."

"I am really trying Sue," I confessed. "But it is really hard for me." Sue just smiled and started the car.

When we drove into the driveway and opened up the car doors, all we could hear were the sounds of buzzing saws. "Brandon is still working diligently," Sue admitted. "Try and get him to take a break every now and then Sue, please."

"I'll watch him," she promised. We entered the house and I started up the stairs. Sue stopped and said, "I am going to see if I can get him to at least have a cup of coffee and take a short break."

"You go on upstairs, I'll be right there," she said. "Okay," I agreed, and I started for the top of the stairs. Once I reached the top, I took a few cleansing deep breaths. The treatments had really begun to take the wind out of my sails. I waited a minute or two and turned for the kitchen. My pain was in full bloom at this moment and I knew that I could no longer put off taking the medication. I walked to the kitchen table not looking to my left, but only concentrating on finding my pills in my purse. I put my purse on the table and began searching for my pain pills. Suddenly out of the corner of my eye, I saw a figure stand and move toward me. I turned and saw my brother.

"Edward," I yelled. I froze right in my tracks and dropped my purse on the floor. He walked up to me and put his arms around me. "Oh Edward, I have missed you so much," I said with my voice cracking and my eyes filling with tears." I hugged him as I have never hugged my brother. "I have really missed you," and now I was sobbing. I have missed you too, little sister. I am here now, he said emotionally. "I shall always be here for you anytime you need me. Just tell me and I will come. he said with tears in his eyes. I am your big brother, and I shall always look out for you. I love you, and always have little sister," he said tenderly.

Chapter 42
Getting Reacquainted

Poor Fern, She was on the couch and I hadn't even noticed her. Once my eyes cleared and my emotions calmed down, I saw her sitting there patiently not saying a word. "Oh Fern, I am so sorry, forgive me. I didn't even see you, I confessed. She smiled and said, "come over here and sit by me and tell me everything. Did you forget that I am still a nurse? I might have a little more insight into all this business than your brother," she said teasingly. I gave her a hug along with the short version of my tale of woe. "It appears like the doctors are definitely on the right track if there are already signs of improvement regarding the tumor. But you do look terrible Pam, and you are so thin." Fern was never the one to mince words. She always spoke her mind whether you wanted to hear her opinion or not. "Are the side effects of the chemo and radiation causing you to lose weight this quickly?" she asked.

"No, unfortunately I had been losing weight a long time before I was diagnosed with cancer. I had been to some specialists, but they missed the cancer and thought that I was just under too much stress." Fern looked a little upset, "well, exactly how long is a long time?" she asked.

"Over a year, and I know what your thinking. But I am on the right track now, and I am going to beat this cancer." I said defiantly.

We heard a voice yelling from the bottom of the stairs. It was Sue. "Can Brandon and I come up stairs now? Is the reunion over?"she asked jokingly.

"Yes, come up and join us," I said cheerfully. Both Brandon and Sue entered the living room smiling. "Sue, you little devil, you knew all along that

Edward and Fern were here when you picked me up from the doctors this morning," I said scolding her.

"I did?" she said laughingly.

Brandon turned and spoke to my brother, "Would you like to see what your money bought Ed, it's right downstairs? I have been working on it, that is where all the noise is coming from."

"Hell yes!," my brother answered. The two of walked out of the room and headed for the downstairs area.

"How much has Brandon accomplished?" Fern asked.

I smiled and admitted, "I'm not allowed downstairs when he is working. I make him crazy, apparently." Fern laughed and said, "Just leave him alone and he'll do fine." Fern changed the subject and asked, "How's the rest of the family doing, and how are they dealing with your illness?"

"Actually, I think they are managing extremely well," I commented.

Sue voiced her opinion, "Most of them are in denial, but they are trying to cope. The realization of the cancer is something that none of us want to face. What would we all do, without Pam?"

I smiled, "You would all do fine. There is nothing that couldn't be handled if you faced it together. I have confidence in all of you. Besides, I plan on getting well and concentrating on doing some of the things I have always dreamed about doing. Of course, I am not sure exactly how long that is going to take, but I willing to wait until my health returns."

Fern and I joined Sue at the kitchen table for some coffee and pastry. I reached down and picked up my purse that I had dropped earlier. It was definitely time for a pain pill. Fern saw me and asked, "Can I see what the doctor has prescribed for you?"

"Sure," I said handing her the bottle.

"Is there more than just this one?" she asked.

"Oh my yes," I said. I reached down into my purse and pulled out the four other bottles of pills. Quite a collection of medications don't you think?" I asked.

Fern admitted, "I've seen a lot more than these prescribed for your condition. Are they helping any of your symptoms?"

"They seem to be, especially the medications for vomiting and diarrhea," I said smiling.

"How often do you go for chemo and radiation treatments?" Fern asked. I explained to her how the chemo was only once a week and the radiation was every day. "Do you have any idea how long you have to endure these treatments? Did the doctors give you any hint of the duration of time?" Fern questioned.

"No, not really, I confessed. I'll just have to go with the flow as the saying goes. What time frame would you guess, Fern?" I asked.

"It's not something I would bet on, but I would estimate at least six or seven months to be on the safe side." she said frowning. My heart sank. How was I ever going to withstand that length of time, feeling the way I do? I tried not to let my disappointment show in my face, but I know both Sue and Fern could read my expression

Brandon and Edward returned from the inspection of the downstairs equipment. Edward spoke first, "Pam you are going to have a nice place to live when Brandon finishes the apartment. He is doing a heck of a job and knows exactly what he is doing."

Brandon smiled, " Some things might take me a little longer than a professional carpenter, but after a while I can usually figure out what I am doing wrong."

Pam, do you feel like going for a short ride?" my brother asked.

"I guess so, as long as it's not to far." I said bravely.

"No, I just need to pick up a few things I had forgotten to get for the bathroom," Brandon admitted. "Okay, lets go then." was my reply.

It was then decided that we would go in Edwards' and Ferns' car as it was a much larger vehicle than what Sue and Bran owned. Edward had parked it in the vacant lot two houses down from Brandon's so that I would not see it when I arrived home that morning. We drove past the radiation building, which I pointed out, and continued to the main street named Post Road. Fairfield was a large city for the state of RI and Post Rd. practically covered one end of Fairfield to the other end of the city. The mall was located on this road as was many other types of business. I did guess that we were probably headed for a large lumber company that supplied all varieties of building equipment.

When Edward pulled into the parking lot of the lumber company, I was not surprised at all. What did surprise me was Edward asked me if I wanted to go inside. "No, not really," I confessed I'll just sit out here in the car and wait." Fern decided to wait with me while Edward, Brandon and Sue went inside. Fern and I chatted about her family in Canada. They were planning to go visit her sister when they left Rhode Island on Sunday. Fern admitted that it had been years since she had seen her family as well.

Before long I saw the family leaving the lumber building. None of them were carrying anything, and I said to Fern, "it looks as if Brandon could not find what he needed for downstairs. I think there is another plumbing supply company a little further down the road from here. We can try that place next."

"No luck finding what you wanted Brandon?" I asked.

"Oh they had what I wanted but it has to be delivered."

"Delivered?" I said confused.

"Yes delivered," Edward answered. "We couldn't carry dry wall in our hands."

"Dry wall?" another stupid question on my part.

"Mom, Edward purchased all the dry wall necessary to complete your entire apartment." Brandon said proudly. I was not able to get a sound out of my mouth. My eyes filled with tears and I placed my head down on Ferns shoulder.

I could hear my brother saying, "Oh here she goes again, crying. She always used to get me in trouble with our Mom by crying." I looked up at him at started to laugh. I have such a wonderful brother.

Chapter 43
Visits

It was then decided that we should return Brandon and Sue to their home and continue on to my Mom and Dads house. "I need to go into the house for a bathroom trip before we continue on, I told my brother. I'll only be a minute," I said as I opened the back door of the car. Brandon, Sue and I went inside while Edward and Fern waited out in the car.

"That is some brother you have Mom," Brandon commented.

"I know. He has always had a kind and generous way. I only wish that we could have spent more time

together. Learn from my mistakes Brandon, appreciate your brother and sister because in this life you never know what will happen from one minute to the next."

"I had never been able to understand why you and Jay are so distant from each other. I realize that your father did tremendous damage to you both, but you are adults now. "omeday after I am dead and gone, Jay and Robin will be all you have left of our little family."

Brandon gave me a sad look and said, "Mom, I have tried over and over to get Jay to come and visit, but he keeps his distance. He is very strange that way, and I have never done anything to cause him to dislike me."

"It is not anything that you have done, Brandon. It's what your father did. He created envy and jealousy between Jay and you. I can't go into it right now because they are waiting for me in the car, but this conversation is to be continued. I better get into the bathroom and back to the car before they decide to leave me," I teased as I hurried up the stairway.

Dad was just coming out of his front door when we drove up to their apartment. A big smile crossed Dad's face once he recognized who was in the car. Edwards first comment when he saw our father walking toward us was, "He never changes no matter how old he gets."

"I know, we were blessed with a good man as our father."

Edward smiled and said, "I'll say."

Dad's first words were, "I'll be damned. Look who finally came home to visit." Dad walked up to Edward and gave him a hug. "It's good to see you Ed."

"I know that it's been a long time Dad, but you know how things are." Edward replied smiling. "How's Mom?"

Dad laughed, "She never changes, she is inside. Go in and surprise her." Dad said hello to Fern and explained that he was just on his way to the market. "I'll be right back, go on inside. I'll get something for your mother to cook for dinner."

Edward shook his head no and replied, "No dad that's not necessary, I'm going to take you and Mom out for lunch."

"Great" dad said. "I'll be back in a couple of minutes."

We rang the door bell and Mom's voice came over the intercom, "Whose there?"

"It's your long lost son, Ed. Are you going to let me in?"

"Oh my God, Edward!" We heard the buzzer sound and the door lock released. Edward looked at me and smiled, "Get ready, here we go."

Mom was all smiles when we walked inside. I knew that it would do her heart good to see Edward. My mother always loved him so much. He could charm her so easily, and looking back, I think that he reminded her of our biological father. Not necessarily in looks, but in his mannerisms. I remember thinking when I was a small child, I wish I could get away with everything my brother does. I was the obedient little girl, and Edward was the devilish little boy who did whatever he wanted and always escaped any discipline.

We sat an talked for about an hour. Edward told Mom of his plans to take us all out for lunch. There is one food in Rhode Island that my brother truly enjoys. That food is known as simply the "Hot Weiner." Apparently, they are not available in other states and, therefore, whenever Edward visits home, he never misses purchasing those "Hot Weiner's" covered with sauce, mustard and onions. There is a small diner not far from our parents apartment that serves those "Hot Weiner's...." We all knew that would be Ed's restaurant of choice.

During lunch we reminisced about when we were kids, reliving some of life's better times. We had a wonderful childhood, and never knew that we were poor. As far as we were concerned, we had everything we wanted and needed. We even spoke of not having a bathroom in our little home, as we lived in an old garage that had been remodeled into a tiny house. There was an old fashioned pump at the sink, and a large cast iron stove in the kitchen that served as a heating system as well as the cook stove. But to us it was home, and we were happy and healthy.

Edward and I started laughing about something silly while we were sitting at the diner. Of course that triggered our mother's usual reaction of disgust. Mom was such an easy target for teasing, as she could never quite understand why we were laughing. The more disgusted she became with us, the more we laughed. "Honestly, you two will never grow up," she stated. "Anyone would think that you were nuts." That statement only caused more laughter on our part. Dad and Fern just sat there and let Edward and myself make fools of ourselves. But we didn't care, we were together and having fun.

After lunch it was time to go and visit Rah and her family. Edward promised Mom that he would return tomorrow to see her again. We drove them to their apartment and then we were on the road again. I was beginning to get very tired and those hot Weiner's were taking their toll on my stomach. It was a very lucky thing for me that Rah's house was practically just around the corner.

Tawnee was the first one out the door when we pulled into their driveway. She was quickly followed by Kyle (name) and then Haley. Rah's children had not seen Edward since they were very young, and their immediate reaction to Edward was a cautious one. Rah had always been very fond of Edward. She had been the target of his teasing when she was a child, and as a result was used to him. Edward could brighten any ones day and usually did where ever he went.

Rah's children were totally drawn to Edward. They sat and listened to every word he said. Tawnee was so cute, she came up to me and whispered, " are you sure he is really your brother?" I laughed loud enough to have Rah ask me what Tawnee had just said to me. I didn't want to embarrass Tawnee (she is an overly sensitive child) so I simply replied "nothing special, I am just very happy today." A smile of relief came over Tawnee's face. I returned her smile and added a wink. The same thought came to my mind again, I can't help but see Rah when I look at Tawnee. I don't think I have ever seen a child resemble her mother as much as she does.

We remained another hour at Rah's and then decided it was time to leave.

Mainly because I fell asleep sitting in an upright position. I don't know what the conversation was while I was asleep, but I am sure it was in regards to my illness. Edward and Fern hugged all the kids goodbye, and once again we were traveling the roads for the return trip to Fairfield.

It was almost to three o'clock when we returned back to Brandon's. Now it was Alex and Bri's turn to see their Uncle Edward. The girls had just came home from school. Once we settled down in the living room and began to talk the girls began their staring. I don't think they meant to be rude; I just believe they were fascinated by Edward. My brother ignored them for a brief time, and then began the all to familiar routine of teasing. Edward called Alex over to him. She came over to him but very shyly, and stood in front of him. To describe my brothers appearance is not an easy task. I have to compare him to a tall birch tree, but heavier around the middle. He is very tall and a white horse shoe shape of hair around his head. He is what most people would describe politely as a "big man." Picture little Alex standing very bravely and asking softly, "Yes?"

My brother looked down at her and seriously said, "Alex I have both my hands behind my back containing some money. In one hand I have a one dollar bill, in the other hand I have a fifty dollar bill. You pick one and which ever one you choose is yours to keep." Alex looked at her father and mother and they both gave her the desired go ahead nod. Alex pointed to his right side and Edward brought his arm in front of him and opened his hand. There it was, a fifty dollar bill! Alex jumped up and down with excitement but did not touch the money. Edward said to her, "go ahead, you picked it. It's yours to keep." Her little hand reached up and swiftly grabbed the fifty dollar bill.

"Thank you, Uncle Edward" she exclaimed, and as quickly as her two feet would carry her she was sitting next to her father. While all this was occurring little Bri was standing quietly in the corner of the kitchen watching. Bri was two years younger than Alex, and had no concept of money nor could she read numbers.

Edward spoke again only calling Bri this time, "Bri would you come over here?" She marched over to Edward, walking straight as an arrow with her little head held high. Edward looked down at her and said, "It's your turn now."

"I know," she answered.

My brother placed a one dollar bill in his left hand and a hundred dollar bill in his right hand. He opened up his hands showing her the money on each palm of his hands. "You may have which ever bill you chose, but you may not change your mind, once you have picked the one you want. Do you understand, Bri?" Edward asked her.

"Yes, I do. I just have to pick one," she said smiling.

"You cannot ask your Mom or Dad which one to pick, the choice is totally up to you," Edward advised her.

"Okay, I can do this by myself." she said proudly.

Edward smiled and said, "Okay then Bri, pick one." Bri stood there for only a few seconds and reached for the hundred dollar bill and politely took it out of his hand. Edward sat there and then started to laugh. "She may be only a tiny little girl, but she sure knows money." Laughter filled the room.

Bri turned around and looked at her father and asked, "Did I pick the good one?"

Brandon answered her as soon as he could stop laughing. "Yes, my little Bri Bri, You picked the good one."

I had to determine why she picked the hundred dollar bill, and so I asked her. "Why did you chose that one Bri?"

"Because I liked the mans face." she replied. Laughter again sounded all through the house.

Excitement filled the living room. Both girls were thrilled to death by their newly acquired wealth. "What are you going to do with all that money?" I asked both girls.

Bri replied, "She was going to buy a turtle.

Alex said, "I am going to save it for your doctor bills, Meme."

The room grew suddenly silent. I reached over and pulled Alex to me kissing her and said, "Alley Cat, you don't have to do that. Meme has very good medical insurance that pays for all her doctor bills. You take the money and buy something very special for yourself."

Edward stood up and stated, " Time to eat! Alex and Bri, you choose the place." The decision was made quickly.

"The Buffet Palace," they both yelled. The rest of us adults were relieved, as we were sure that we would be eating in a hamburger place with the girls being allowed to make the choice. I would have preferred to send them on their way and stay home and lie down, but how often was I going to get the chance to be with my brother. So when none of them were paying any attention, I slipped another pain pill in my mouth and hoped that it would start doing it's job as rapidly as possible.

Sue and Fern reached for their pocketbooks and Brandon and Edward got the coats for Alex and Bri. Once again we were headed for the car. I thought to myself, it has been a long, long wonderful day. Thank you God!

Chapter 44
Bathroom Completion

The dinner, as anticipated, was wonderful at the Buffet Palace. Of course I knew that it was the company, not food that made everything so nice. We sat there a long time after we had finished eating just talking and enjoying being together. I kept looking at all of us at the table, it was so nice to be surrounded by people that you love.

I was tired by the time we returned home, and I had to go to bed almost immediately. I hated to leave Edward and Fern, but I knew that Brandon and Sue would entertain them in my absence. I had over indulged myself in every way possible today, and now I was paying for it. I excused myself from my family and went into the girls bedroom and shut the door. I barely remember getting undressed. I think I fell asleep instantly when my head hit the pillow. I had to get up only once in the middle of the night. It was nice having the bathroom so close. I remember thinking, where am I tonight? I hadn't realized it, but Alex was in the bed with me. Bri must have been told to sleep with her Mom and Dad to give me extra room in their regular size bed.

The voices coming from the kitchen must have awakened me. I recognized Sue's voice and then I heard Fern speaking, as one cannot mistake that French accent. *I could also smell food cooking*, and *I thought, oh I am not hungry at all. I hope that no one insists that I eat a big breakfast this morning. I don't think my stomach could handle it. I definitely don't want to start vomiting with my brother here, and the last thing I want Edward to remember about this visit is his sister throwing up.*

I gathered up my strength and walked out into th kitchen. Fern immediately asked, "Pam, how are you feeling this morning?"

"A little better, but I still feel tired. Can you believe that?" I asked.

"That is perfectly normal, and it is going to get a lot worse before it gets better Pam," Fern advised. "That's a happy thought," I said trying to smile.

"You'll get through it, just take it day by day," Fern said.

"I don't think I am going to be very good company today for you and my brother. Why don't you take this opportunity and visit some of your old friends that you haven't seen in a long time?" I suggested. I know my brother, and I am sure he wouldn't want to pass up the opportunity to see old friends. The last thing I want you to do is sit and watch me sleep all day," I admitted.

"You over exerted yesterday, didn't you?" Sue stated.

"A little, but it was worth it to me. I enjoyed every second of the day, and I would do it again today, if I were physically able." While we sat there talking, Edward came upstairs. He didn't appear as if he had just awakened. "I thought you were still sleeping?" I asked.

"No, I wasn't sleeping, I was assisting the plumber downstairs. He needed my expertise," Edward said jokingly.

"Oh God, now the toilet will never work!" I teased.

"Very funny, little sister, but you would be surprised how much I know about pipes and water fixtures," he stated confidently. "It's only a matter of time before your little bathroom is totally finished and working properly. Pam, your son is an excellent plumber, as well as a great mechanic," Edward said being very complimentary. "In fact, if no one minds, I am headed for where he works right now to have them check my brakes and an oil change for the preparation of the trip to Canada and then the return trip back home again, Edward admitted. Plus all it's going to cost me is an iced coffee for the guys that work there. Brandon made a phone call and set it up for me. The guys are waiting for me to get there right now, if no one minds?"

"Don't be silly Edward, go an get it done," I assured him.

"Pam is too tired to do much of anything today. She over did yesterday, and she wants you and Fern to go an enjoy yourself by visiting some of your Rhode Island friends while you have the opportunity," Sue replied.

Edward mulled this one over for a minute, and then confirmed the idea with Fern, "What do think hun?" "Sounds like fun to me, let's do it," she replied.

"Good, I said. It's settled."

"Well I will see you later on, I have to get back to work or my mother will nag me," Brandon teased. Edward turned to Fern and asked, "Why don't you come with me, your dressed, and we can leave from the car repair shop?"

"Okay, I'll just get my purse," Fern replied. Are you sure you don't mind?" she asked me.

I shook my head no and said, "Just go and enjoy yourself. But make sure your are back by five o'clock."

"I am making my special spaghetti for supper," Sue advised. "I did talk to Jays early this morning early and he and Ann shall be joining us for supper." He wants to see you and Fern also," Sue said smiling. Edward smiled and said, "Great, I haven't had the chance to see their little girl, what's her name?"

I answered, "Cheyenne."

"Okay then we will be on our way and shall return by five o'clock. See you then." Fern said. They walked down the stairs and headed for the front door.

"Edward?" I yelled. Don't forget to stop in and see Mom and Dad again today. Mom will be very upset if you don't. Especially because you are leaving tomorrow morning so early, so please stop in there if only for a few minutes. It will make her happy," I pleaded.

"I will, so stop worrying little sister, bye for now," and they walked out the front door.

I spent the rest of the day just lying on the bed or the couch. I was really feeling out of it today. I think that today has been the worst as far as my lack of strength. I could hear Brandon working away all day. His friends stopped in and stayed for about two hours downstairs with him. I hope they were helping him, but knowing Brandon as I do, he would have probably liked working alone better than with inexperienced carpenters. Rah called around three o'clock just checking on everyone. She apologized for not coming over, but she knew there was enough confusion going on and by her staying home with her family it made things easier for me and Sue. Rah also confirmed with me that she would pick me up tomorrow afternoon in preparation for the Monday morning chemo treatment.

Alex and Bri had spent the day at Sue's mothers house to keep them out of their fathers hair downstairs while he was working. I kind of missed the little ones. They had such a positive effect on me. They were just so loving and caring. They could always maneuver to make me smile no matter how badly I was feeling. Sue could tell that I was having a bad day, and she constantly kept checking on me and trying to feed me. I assured her that I was fine, just tired. She didn't have to worry about me so much.

I returned to the bedroom after speaking with Rah on the phone. Monday was not my favorite days, and today my mind was focused on financial matters as well as my physical weakness. I just couldn't come up with any form of improving my financial position. I just don't know how I shall manage without money coming in. Brandon and Sue have just barely enough to make ends meet. Sure, I had made money on the furniture sale, but that money was totally accounted for. There was no one that could help me. My credit was a total disaster, bill collectors were constantly notifying me that they were going to take me to court. My house was gone, my car, and there was no money coming in from the Post Office. I just can't think about it any more.

I lay there on the bed until four o'clock. I knew that I had to get up and showered and dressed before Edward and Fern and the rest of the company arrived. I forced myself to enter the bathroom and began my usual routine. Crying. *Be brave Pam, don't let your brother see you lose it*, I thought. *You can handle it, you can handle anything.* By the time I finished dressing and fixing up, I looked fairly presentable. I walked into the kitchen and Sue saw me.

"Well you do look better, but how do you actually feel?"

"I am a little better but still weak. Perhaps the weakness is the result of yesterday," I said hopefully. "Maybe, Sue replied. Just sit down, I have it all handled."

"The spaghetti smells wonderful Sue," I said inhaling the smell.

Sue smiled, "Well, it's all set to go. I am just waiting for everyone to return. Pam, what's with Jay? I have asked Brandon what the problem is between he and his brother, but he never gives me an answer?" I looked at Sue and shrugged my shoulders, "Sue, I don't think Brandon knows the answer to that question himself."

As we were standing there talking, Brandon came up the stairs. "Mom, I thought I heard your voice. Would you like to come downstairs and see what I have accomplished?"

"Yes, I would love to. Do I have your permission?" I said teasing him.

"Don't be funny, just follow me," he commanded. I walked next to him on the stairway, and when we turned to go into the basement I stopped dead in my tracks. The entire basement was totally dry walled into separate rooms. I could see the metal strips on the ceiling that were awaiting the ceiling tiles to be placed inside them. "Come on Mom, there is a lot more to see," Brandon stated. I know that I must have looked shocked, because I was. There were two more doors added as we walked down the small hallway. I recognized my bedroom door, but the other two were newly added additions. Brandon opened the first door to my left, it led into the laundry room, the second door I knew was my bathroom. "You open it Mom," Brandon suggested. I held my breath and opened the door. What I saw was a totally completed bathroom with all the fixtures in working condition. He had the shower running, the sink faucet had running water coming out of it, and all the lights were turned on. Everything was in place. My bathroom vanity and mirror were installed, along with electrical outlets all placed in the proper areas for use. "Mom, you flush it first," he said laughing. I placed my hand on the little handle, pushed down gently, and the water started to swirl and flush. "It all works perfectly, and there all no leaks."

"You are all set now Mom, there shall be no more walking up and down the stairs in the middle of the night."

"Brandon, you did all this yourself in two days?"I asked.

"I had a little help from my friends, but yes, I did mostly by myself. Do you like it?" he asked.

"Like it, I love it. Thank you son," and I threw my arms around him and hugged him with all my strength.

Chapter 45
Dinner for 10

The different families arrived approximately within ten minutes of each other. The first family members were Edward and Fern, followed by Jay and Ann who was holding Cheyenne. Greetings, and hugs were followed by general conversation. Edward and Fern properly admired little Cheyenne's beauty, as she looked adorable dressed in a little pink outfit. Alex and Bri could not keep their hands off her. That just had to hold her. Ann gave her permission, with the condition that they would only hold here while they were seated. That was just a precaution that she did not get accidently dropped. Cheyenne just smiled, and cooed at them and made her usual gurgling sounds.

Edward and Jay were escorted downstairs by Brandon to show off his carpentry skills. Jay was very impressed with his brothers abilities. I sat in the kitchen wishing that Rah could have been here with her family as well. Had she been, there the family picture would have been completed.

Sue had worked long and hard on this dinner, everything was ready and she would accept absolutely no assistance from anyone. The conversation over dinner was kept light and humorous. Even stern faced Jay had to laugh out loud at some of Edward's jokes.

Edward and Fern talked of their day visiting old friends. They truly enjoyed themselves. I am not sure of the number of people that they visited, but I am almost positive there were least three different families they had visited. Edward advised me he kept his promise, and stopped and visited Mom and Dad. That pleased me very much, as I am sure that Mom and Dad were happy about their visit as well. Who knows when they will see them again? Edward told them that he and Fern would be leaving first thing in the morning, but he promised them he would keep in touch.

I kept the conversation on different subjects staying clear of any mention of my cancer. But, unfortunately Jay and Ann wanted to be filled in on exactly the prognosis. They inquired about my last visit to the doctor and what was said. Jay stated that if he was to ever get cancer he would never take chemo treatments. That left an opening for Edward to give him a classic insult. Edward could not resist asking Jay this question, "Why wouldn't you go for chemo treatments, you have already lost your hair!" Of course that little insult caused my brother to laugh out loud at his own joke. Jay, on the other hand, failed to appreciate the humor in Edwards's statement.

Jay's was smiling, but his reply was, "Funny Edward, very funny. I do not appreciate the humor in that statement dear Uncle. At least I had hair on my head longer than you. I didn't lose my hair until I was twenty one. How old were you? Mom said you were only around nineteen when your hair had totally vanished," he asked with a smirk.

"Oh no you don't you two, I am not going to get caught in the middle of this little go-around, "I replied laughing. I am not saying a word regarding hair. Still laughing I said, "Mine is still here and I am hoping that it will stay that way."

After the meal the family returned to the living room for more reminiscing. Edward and I spoke about our childhood and how he would always tell me that I was adopted. Bran followed with how he and Jay would tease each other, and how I had purchased a pair of boxing gloves for them to get out their frustrations. We all had different stories that stuck in our minds and repeated them to jog each others memories. Laughter filled the room.

Jay talked about his work and being a new father. Ann remained quiet, as was her usual manner, and held the baby. Edward talked about traveling with Fern and just enjoying life.

Sue changed the subject asking, "Does anyone want desert?" Of course no one refused, and so the conversations continued for a while longer over desert and coffee.

The time flew by quickly and it became quite late. Jay and Ann had a long drive back to Connecticut so they were the first to leave. Jay promised to keep in touch with Edward, and also promised not to be such a stranger at his brothers house. Edward, of course, invited everyone to come and visit he and Fern when ever they wished to. My home is open to anyone of you, or all of you at the same time," he announced proudly. Laughing, he added, "The trick is to find where I am living, because I don't know where Fern and I will be from one day to the next." Naturally everyone promised they would stay in contact with each other, but I know that won't happen. As much as I wish my family would stay close with one other, I feel there is something that prevents them from achieving that goal.

I was feeling terribly exhausted, and could have fallen asleep standing up, but I wanted to spend as much time with my brother as possible. I knew that Edward had planned to leave as early in the morning as they could (around 6 a.m.). I thought, *who knows how long it will be before I see him and Fern again. If I am lucky, perhaps a year, or two? I truly hope that after this cancer business is finished, I could go and visit them for a couple of weeks. But time will tell.*

Bran, Sue and I stayed up talking with Ed and Fern until after 11 p.m. Fern was tired and stated she was not looking forward to the long drive to Canada. "You must excuse me, but I really must get some sleep," Fern stated. She reaffirmed her thoughts regarding my cancer and attempted to comfort me by saying, "You are going to make it through this with flying colors, Pam. I know because I am a nurse, she said smiling. Just stay positive, and keep in touch. If you need us, we are only a

phone call away no matter where we are living." I hugged her and thanked her for everything she and Edward had done for me.

"Someday, I shall repay you for all your kindness," I stated crying.

"Don't concern yourself with that. Just get better and make sure you call and let us know how you are doing," Fern requested. She turned and walked downstairs. On her way down the stairs she yelled, Edward, don't stay up much later. It's a long drive."

"Okay hun," I will be down in a minute or two and go to bed." Edward and I spoke about Mom and Dad and how he does worry about them. "But there is nothing I can do for them." he stated.

I told him not to worry that I would look out for them. " I am here in Rhode Island, and I am in touch with them everyday Edward." I said trying to comfort him.

"Pam, you take care of yourself. They are both healthier than you are," he said.

"I know that Edward, but I don't want you to worry them. I keep them at a distance as far as my health is concerned, I admitted. You know how Mom worries," I said. Edward had a concerned look on his face and finally said, "I am going to say it again to you Pam, take care of yourself right now. Promise me right now Pam," he said. Promise me that you will call me anytime you need me."

"Okay, I promise," I said with tears in my eyes. I leaned over and hugged my brother and told him, "I love you."

He returned my hug and admitted, "I love you too little sister. Now go to bed and get some rest, and I will be calling you regularly to check on you," he confessed.

Edward said good night to everyone and thanked Bran and Sue for their hospitality and went down stairs. God I loved my brother, and I had never realized how much until this moment. I wanted to cry so badly, my tears were almost there, but I held them back. I didn't want anyone to see me cry. I walked into the bedroom, undressed and said my prayers. I wanted to remember everything about my brothers visit and keep it in my hear forever. I lay there and gave thanks for the wonderful day I had just experienced. I only wished that my daughter could have been there with her family to complete my happiness.

Today was Sunday, and Edward and Fern had departed for their trip to Canada. Edward had placed a note for me on my vanity. It was his cell phone number. All the note said was "to be called anytime his little sister needed help." The note brought a large smile on my face and the all to familiar lump in my throat. Oh no, not today I thought to myself. Today I am taking my very first shower in my personal new bathroom. I will not cry today.

It was becoming very difficult to hide the fact that my weakness was getting worse. I felt as if my life was being drained right out of my body. Sometimes it was extremely difficult just to hold up my head. My body craved sleep. It did not matter how many hours a day that I slept, I always seemed to need more. Fern had stated that it was going to get worse before it got better and she was correct in her observation. I wondered how I was going to get through all these future treatments? The holidays were approaching fast. Thanksgiving was only a week away. I couldn't ever bear to think about Christmas. Just the sight of an advertisement on tv regarding Christmas would send me into a panic attack. I had absolutely no money and there was going to be none coming. I had considered calling Social Security and the RI Welfare Department. Perhaps there was a chance that one of those choices would be able to assist me in my time of need. I thought, *I will call one or both of them this week. I will also ask Sue about the Welfare system. She was raised on welfare. There were six children in her family and her father was unable to work.*

If anyone can help me with questions, it will be Sue. Welfare was not something I wanted to do. I still had pride. I had worked all my life and never asked for assistance from anyone. Just the thought of having to apply for food stamps was causing me heart ache and shame. But I was in a position were beggars cannot be choosers. God help me and give me strength. I know the good Lord does not approve in pride. So I shall swallow mine and attempt to ask for help.

Rah arrived with my granddaughters Tawnee and Haley. I thought Alex and Bri would faint from excitement. Every time those four little girls saw each other it was as they hadn't seen each other in years. The two older girls, Tawnee and Alex, would pair off leaving the younger two, Haley and Bri to play by themselves. But it usually worked out for the best and they played their separate little games and had a wonderful time.

"I'm sorry that I could not be here yesterday Mom, but there were enough people here to fill a stadium, and I didn't think you need any more additions to the visitors list," she said with a large smile. "How did it go? Did everyone have a good time? I need to know, tell me all about it," she said inquisitively.

I told her, "Everything went very nicely and she and her family were missed by everyone."

"Well, I have been thinking about Thanksgiving dinner, and I would like everyone to come to my house this year," Rah said smiling.

I replied, "Are you sure, that is a lot of people Rah?"

"Not to worry Mom, I can handle it. Besides, Sue will help me, won't you Sue?"

Sue's reply was a simple, "of course."

"I want to have a dinner just like the ones you made every year at Thanksgiving. We will make this a real celebration and give thanks for your cancer getting better, " Rah said with assurance in her voice.

"I won't be able to help much," I confessed.

Rah just gave me one of her, I'll handle it looks and pretended I didn't say anything at all. "So it's settled then, and I will get working on it right away," Rah said proudly.

Chapter 46
Routine Residence Change

I took my change of clothes that I had packed for my Monday treatment day. My prescriptions were tucked away in the bottom of my pocketbook for safe keeping. I said my good byes to Bran and Sue and gave kisses and hugs to Alex and Bri and I was once again on the road.

I struggled with staying awake while in route to Rah's house. I had not taken my pain medication as my pain did not warrant any. I had also followed Dr. Merrick's instructions regarding writing down exactly how long of a period of time it was between pain medication. I was dreading tomorrow morning. Mondays were so difficult on me. As each Monday passed it became more and more draining. I didn't want to complain, but I knew that when I arrived at Rah's home, I was going have to lie down and get some sleep. I would watch the kids play Nintendo. They enjoyed playing the game so much, and then explaining to me how to move from one level to the next and retrieve the coveted stars as the award. It was such a small thing that they wanted from me, and I found the music to their little game very soothing. I didn't mind watching them. It made me feel wanted and not a burden to my Rah.

Greg was home waiting for the arrival of his wonderful mother-in-law. I love to tease him, always reminding him how fortunate he is to have me for his mother-in-law. But Greg has a good since of humor and takes my little jokes very nicely. He was standing in the front door as we pulled into the driveway. He immediately opened the door and said, "Hi Meme."

"Do you have a suitcase you need me to carry?"

I answered, "No Greg, I only have a small overnight bag and the kids can carry it. You only have to put up with me for one night. So you can relax," I said teasing.

He noticed that I was slightly shaky on my feet and immediately came out the door to assist me into the house. Greg spoke while assisting me, "You over did when your brother was here, didn't you?"

I replied with a sigh, "Yes, I did, but we had such a wonderful time being together."

When Greg finally managed to get me to the couch in the living room he said, "Meme why don't you just lie back and try to rest?"

"She really out did herself this weekend, and now she is paying for it big time!" Rah sputtered. Rah instructed the kids to play in their rooms or outside and let me sleep. If I hadn't felt so poorly, I would not of allowed her to send the children away. But I was just so very tired. I couldn't even argue. I will make it up to the kids when I wake up. Perhaps I will feel stronger then.

I woke to the sounds of plates clinking in the kitchen. " Is that you Rah?" I asked sleepily.

"Your awake Mom?" she answered. I didn't mean to wake you."

"That's okay, I needed to wake up. I will never sleep good tonight, if I sleep the entire day away." The children were sitting on the love seat and the floor being very, very quiet. "My goodness, I didn't even realize that you little ones were in the room, I said smiling at all of them. Thank you for being so good and letting your old Meme sleep." Big smiles immediately appeared on all of their faces. "How about a game of Mario before your mother says dinner is ready?"

"Yeah!" they all yelled. And the game began.

I watched the children play for almost an half and hour before Rah announced the dinner was served. I never realized that Rah was such a good cook. I managed to get Tawnee to pull me up from the couch.

"Mom you stay where you are, I will bring the food to you," Rah said sternly.

"No, I have to move around some. I think my body needs some exercise or I will become weaker and weaker. Tawnee will help me to the table, so stop worrying."

I did my best to try and act perfectly normal sitting at the table. I tried to show that I was not in any discomfort. Silly me, Rah had me figured down to the letter.

"Mom, you are really hurting aren't you? Where is the pain?"she asked.

"It's in the lower region Rah. The radiation is really doing a number on my skin. I feel like I am burned to a crisp," I confessed.

"I'll talk to the doctor tomorrow about it Mom," she said. "Please try and eat a little more. You hardly have eaten ten bites. I'm worried about your eating habits. You can't stay strong if you don't eat." she said in her firmest voice.

"I know, but I just can't swallow it Rah. It's seems to get stuck in my throat," I answered.

She just shook her head and said, "I will bring that up tomorrow at the doctors as well."

Tawnee and Rah began to clear off the dishes from the dinner table. "I feel so helpless," I confessed.

"Well that is just too bad for you," Rah said teasing.

"We can handle it Meme," Tawnee replied. So there I sat watching them both move around the kitchen like lightning bolts. Rah never skipped a beat. If she was interrupted by one of the kids or Greg, she never changed her pace. She was amazing to watch. *Naturally, I took credit* and thought, *I've taught her well.*

Rah was a terrific mother and her children loved her madly. She kept everything running smoothly and appeared to have it all together. But I knew better, I was her mother. She was scared to death about me. I was so proud of her. She had grown into a wonderful woman. Not every mother can say that about their daughter and would be telling the truth. But I am. She is a wonderful daughter, a great mother, and a loving wife. Rah had many struggles in her early life, which I will not go into at this point. But she made it through everything. She is a very strong woman and has proved it on many occasions.

The whole family returned to the living room and began to watch some movie that was playing on the tv. I was beginning to get sleepy again, but I kept forcing myself to stay awake. I lasted until approximately nine o'clock, and that is when Rah sent the kids to bed. I fell asleep almost immediately once the room became child less.

I awoke with severe discomfort and made my way into the kitchen for some water to take one of my pills. I had no idea what time it was as my eyes had not focused on the clock. Rah walked out of the bedroom and looked surprised to see me standing there. "I couldn't sleep any longer Rah," I said before she could ask.

"Well, I was going to wake you up anyway Mom. It's time for you to get ready to go the doctors."

"Rah I want to ask the doctor today how long the chemo treatment is going to continue." I said firmly. I asked her to remind me to find out the answer to that question at some point during the treatment today even if it meant asking one of the nurses. "Perhaps I will get an exam today by Dr. Johnson. Not that I am looking forward to the good old stirrups, but I would like to know what his opinion is regarding my tumor." After I had finished drinking my coffee, I headed for my safe place …the shower. I felt so physically ill and weak I didn't feel as if I could make it through another minute of life. Last night in my dreams my house had been sucked into the ground and I was being chased by men in white and blue uniforms with their hands full of letters. I assume the letters represented bills. Another weird nightmare to chalk up as clearing my mind.

I let the water in the shower spray over me as I sat on the bottom of the tub. I kept thinking, if I die, I will have no money worries. I will be totally free of all the burdens that have been weighing so heavy on me. I can't stand it any more, I just can't take it. Maybe Gods plan is to take me away from all this pain. Dear God, I would go willingly. My only regret would be leaving my family. But in my heart I believe that even in heaven you can watch over the people you love. It would be a gift to them, if I were to die. They would not have to be burdened with me, and they would have some money from my insurance. I started to cry. Not my will ….but thy will.

Rah and I drove to the Women Cancer Center each carrying a coffee. We talked all the way there about the upcoming holiday, Thanksgiving. I was looking forward to spending that day with all my family. It might be my last holiday with them and I was going to fully enjoy it.

The chemo treatment went smoothly but again I did not get the chance to see Dr. Johnson. I asked the nurse, "Do you have any idea how many of these chemo treatments I am scheduled for?"

She replied, "Let me check your chart and I will be right back." Rah and I sat and waited, I had my fingers crossed all the time the nurse was gone. She came back within five minutes and stated, "You are scheduled for treatments until the end of January, if all goes well."

"The end of January?" I said loudly.

"Mom lets go and we will talk about it in the car," Rah said as she squeezed my hand.

223

Chapter 47
Thanksgiving Dinner

The next thirteen days passed by without hardly any recollection on my part. The days were coming and going with only passing moments that I can actually recall. Days were becoming blurry. The weakness and medication were taking their toll on my body. Some days I could only recall a moment or two of the previous day. The only positive side of the situation was that the pain was subsiding more and more every day.

The day that is the most vivid in my mind was late one evening as I lay quietly on the couch. I sat straight up and announced that I had not taken a pain pill the entire day. I had not required one. The pain was gone. My excitement was overwhelming. This could only mean that the tumor was reacting positively to the treatments. I remember saying "Thank you God!" right out loud. The most discomfort I had now was from the radiation. Good grief, was I uncomfortable. But it was nothing compared to the pain I had endured over the past two years. The prescription seemed to help a little for my lower discomfort, but with radiation every day it was like fighting a losing battle. Until the radiation was over with, this condition was going to continue. I was just going to have to deal with it.

I do remember a day last week. (I can't recall exactly what day) but what a day it was. I had called the Social Security Department and requested information regarding a disability claim . The person I talked to on the phone was very pleasant and knowledgeable. The entire application process was completed over the phone. The conversation consisted of an hours worth of questions regarding my work record. When I started work, how long I worked, how much money I made, and so on. After the conversation was finished I was given the wonderful news that if I should be approved, and that's a big if, I had to be out of work six months before I would be eligible for any type of compensation. I thought, well that is really going to help me right now, isn't it. I thanked them for their courtesy, and asked the person what was his recommendations would be for me during the lapse in the time while waiting for their decision. His suggestion was to call the welfare department.

Previously, Sue had called the Welfare department and scheduled an appointment for me to speak with a social worker. After speaking with the Social Security representative on the phone, Sue and I left to speak (in person) with the social worker.

I had gotten myself in a terrible mental condition after the conversation with the Social Security Department, and I should have cancelled the appointment with welfare, but with the money conditions the way they were, I had to force myself to try. At this point, I had nothing to lose but my self esteem. When we arrived at the Welfare Department, I was already crying. It took a few minutes sitting in the car to gather up my courage to go in and speak with the social worker.

We walked in, and I was given several forms to fill out. Once again there were more questions regarding my medical condition, my work records, where I was living, etc. Upon completion of the forms, I was called into a social workers office and sat down in front of her desk. She asked some questions regarding my financial situation, such as if I had a bank account, what kind of car I had and a few other personal facts. I kept myself together the best I could and explained my situation. "I have no money coming in, I cannot collect Temporary Disability Insurance because the Post Office does not take that out of my check every week. Which, makes me ineligible for it. I have no savings, and I have no vacation or sick time left," I said crying. Then I explained to her that I had lost my house and my car because I could not pay for them and up until one month ago, I had no place to live. And as a result of all these things, I was now living at my sons residence.

The woman sat there and looked at me. She pulled open one of her desk drawers and took out a box of Kleenex and handed me one. "I am truly so sorry," she said sincerely. I apologized to her for crying so much, but explained to her that I had always worked, and I had never asked for any help before in my life. "I am so ashamed just to be sitting here," I said. You cannot imagine how devastating this is for me. I am in such a terrible state, and I am sure that you could not understand what I am feeling unless you were in my shoes. I still have my pride and sitting here and asking for help is worse than my cancer." I admitted.

The woman began to figure on the calculator in front of her, and then she just stopped. She looked up at me and said, "I am ashamed to tell you this." She reached for a tissue for herself and her eyes filled with tears. "Ms Ayer, the state can only allow you $26 every two weeks for food. This is because you are living with your son, and because you might be eligible for Social Security, that is the full amount that we can assist you with."

"I don't understand, I said. You help people that come from other countries? I see people all the time with a welfare card, and they don't even speak English." She just sat there and looked at me. "Never mind, just rip up my application and forget that I ever came her for help," I said crying. I stood up from my chair and before she could say another word I walked out of her office. Sue was sitting reading a magazine when I walked into the reception area. "Sue, please get me out of here now!" I requested. She got up out of the chair and assisted me out of the building. I was sobbing. I tried to explain to her what had happened in between the tears.

She was shocked and said, "Pam we are going to manage. Don't get yourself so upset, it will be alright." On the drive home, I told Sue that I did not want anyone to know about what had happened and she promised that she would keep it to her self.

Thanksgiving day was almost here. The weather was following the typical late fall season in New England scenario. The sun was shining, but the temperature was very brisk and chilly. The leaves had already fallen from the trees and were scattered over each and every yard in the neighborhood. New England's weather was special. The weather was famous for changing from one day to the next. No one could ever really plan on what kind of a day was coming. I have celebrated many Thanksgiving Days with the snow flying, and the wind howling. Or, the holiday weather might be warm and sunny. But either type of weather was accepted. Nothing dampens a New England Thanksgiving Day celebration, and that includes the weather. As with every where else in the world, it was a day of giving thanks, and rain, snow, ice or sleet would not ruin family celebrations.

Thanksgiving Day is only two days away. This year I was celebrating it more than I had ever done in my entire life. I was going to enjoy the day with my family, and I was getting a reprieve from my radiation treatments for three days. What more could I ask for. I was like a child in school waiting for the much anticipated holiday vacation. "Thank you God!" was all I kept saying.

Rah had been very busy cooking and preparing for the big day. The house smelled like a restaurant. I wish that I was able to enjoy the food like I used too. I had always had a big appetite and never had a problem putting away a big plate of food. Someday soon, I hope, I will be able to enjoy eating again.

The plan for the big day was for all the families to bring some type of food dish with them. It had been agreed upon between themselves who was bringing what. So, I hoped that everything would go according to plan. I was not kept in the loop, Rah was managing the whole dinner. I just smiled to myself and kept my fingers crossed for her sake that there is no disaster. I realize that Thanksgiving Day will be a long one, and I also realize that it is being done for my sake as well as theirs. They want this dinner as a "just in case" Mom is not around next year. I hate to be quite so morbid, but the truth is the truth. I just want the entire family to know how much they all mean to me and how very much I love them. I am truly looking forward to Thanksgiving Day dinner.

When the day arrived I was more excited than anyone else. Rah had to practically tie me to the couch to keep me out of the kitchen. Each one of my kids came with their families and their food edition to the dinner menu. We sat at different make- shift tables and gave thanks to the Lord. I am pretty sure that it was Haley who said grace. Of course there was a little squabbling regarding who would say the prayer, but it was settled peacefully and said perfectly by little Haley. I sat there at the head of the table admiring my family. I was so proud of them all. They were all good and caring parents with beautiful children. If you asked a mother what she would want from her children, it would be what I received that Thanksgiving Day. Love! They loved me, and they loved their families. I had so much to be thankful for, and I was grateful for the chance to realize it before it could have been taken away from me.

When the feast was through, I was banished into the living room with the grandchildren. The men separated themselves from the females and headed for the nearest tv for the "football games." I sat in the living room with my Mom on one side of me and Tawnee on the other. Tawnee was reading another book. Where ever Tawnee was, she was accompanied by a book. I believed she started reading before she was five years old. She was the "reader" of the family. Alex was the total opposite. She wanted to be a model. The only reading she wanted to do was in a Teen magazine. The younger kids were running around with the usual laughter and arguing. Alex would try her best to entice Tawnee into some girl talk, but little Tawnee usually kept her nose in the book.

"Pam, your looking well today," my Mom admitted.

"I've been trying to get some rest and Rah won't allow me to do anything. I thank you for the complement, but I haven't lost my eye sight yet. I know that your fibbing to me, but I appreciate the effort, I replied smiling. I look like a walking skeleton, but it's only temporary. I'll get my weight back as soon as I finish my treatments," I said with confidence in my voice.

The ladies were busy clearing off the table and doing dishes. The sound of their voices and their laughter were wonderful for me to hear. I had always wanted my family to be close, and this disaster concerning me and my health seems to be pulling the family together. "Whose ready for desert?" Rah yelled out. The sounds of moaning filled the room. "Not me," I answered. "I'm to full right now, maybe in a little while." Unfortunately she received the same reply from almost all of the adults. The children, on the other hand, were ready for the second round of food to be served. Ra had made wonderful cookies, and a pumpkin pie. Ann had made a mince meat pie, and Sue had brought some Italian pastry. There was enough deserts to feed an army.

I remained seated in the living room resting and enjoying the rest of the day. I knew that I had over indulged myself, and that bathroom was going to be visited by me on a steady basis but I did not care. I thought to myself, I will be able to sleep all day tomorrow and the next day if necessary. Nothing was going to spoil this day. I will think about the cancer and the bills,…. tomorrow.

I asked Sue and Bran, "are you guys coming to visit me tomorrow?"

Sue replied, "No, not you won't see us at all this long weekend. We will let you rest the next three days, and I will pick you up Monday afternoon at the radiation building. Take some time and recuperate Pam, I know that you are feeling very weak," Sue said.

"Yes, we all know it Mom, Rah replied.

" No matter how much you try and hide it, none of us are stupid," Brandon added

"Alright, I am going to rest and sleep all weekend. Are you all happy now?" I asked. The reaction was all smiles and the nod of heads. "Good grief!" "I can't win," I said smiling at all of them.

I can barely remember saying good bye to everyone that day. I was exhausted. I had really done nothing physical, but perhaps the excitement was harder on me than I thought it would be. But I was a very happy but very tired woman. It had been a good day.

Chapter 48
Patience Required

During the long three day weekend, I was totally useless. My vomiting had reoccurred and I had absolutely no energy. The medication that I had been taking for the nausea was no longer controlling the vomiting. With each passing day, I had hoped that the nausea would improve. But with each day the vomiting was getting worse. I kept thinking to myself, I can't continue like this. I am losing my patience and my confidence regarding my recovery. I need a positive attitude to recover from this cancer. I have to keep fighting, but it is so hard. I am weakening every day. Please God, give me strength. I must be just like Scarelett . Tomorrow.... I will be better.

Monday morning arrived, Rah and I were once again on the road to the doctors office. "If I should forget to mention my nausea to the nurses, please remind me Rah," I asked.

"I won't forget, don't worry, " Rah replied. As we drove into the parking area, I had to run inside to the nearest ladies room. I barely made it inside the stall door before my early morning coffee came up. I sat there on the floor with a great deal of disgust. "I won't cry," I said out loud. "I will not let this get to me, it is only temporary."

"Mom, are you alright," Rah asked.

"Yes, I am just talking to myself. Just ignore me, I said with the lump in my throat. I will be out in just a second."

I got myself to a standing position and took several deep cleansing breaths. I walked out of the stall and Rah reached for me. "Just get me to the sink. I just need to rinse my mouth and splash some water on my face. I'll be alright in a minute or two, Rah" I said trying to reassure her.

"Mom, I can't stand to see you like this, " Rah confessed.

"I'm getting better Rah. The tumor is shrinking, this is just stupid side effects. Please don't worry."

I said. "Rah, I think that the chemo treatments are in full swing and at the maximum level of dosage. It must be the reason why the medicine is not working any like it used to. Perhaps the doctor can prescribe something stronger for me. When we get upstairs, I intend to talk to one of the nurses regarding my vomiting.

It wasn't long before I was sitting in my familiar chair receiving the chemo through my veins. My hands were one big black and blue mark. All these needles going in and out were leaving their trademarks. About an hour passed of the treatment process, when I started to feel much better. The nausea had ceased and considering that I was receiving chemo, I felt good. I waited until the nurse came in to check on me and then I asked her, "What kind of medicine besides the chemo is in the IV?" "One is a saline solution, the other is an drug for nausea, and of course the chemo," she answered.

"Is it possible to get the drug for nausea in pill form? My nausea has returned and I need something stronger to control it. Whatever is going inside me right now works very well."

"If you don't mind waiting, I will check that out for you. she replied. Do you have good medical coverage?" she asked.

"Yes, my ex-husband works for the State, so the coverage is the best anyone could ask for."

"I will find out what I can for you and get back to you before you are through today. But before I forget, I was told to inform you that after the treatment, Dr Johnson wants to exam you in room #4." she said smiling.

"Gee, that is just what I wanted to hear," I replied with a grimace. She smiled at me and left the room.

Rah was looking at me strangely, and said, "Mom your color looks one hundred times better than when you came in here today."

I smiled and replied, "I feel so much better Rah, you would not believe it." I sat in the chair while the treatment continued for another hour when the nurse came back into the room with a prescription in her hand.

"I checked with Dr. Johnson and he gave me this new prescription for you to try," she said handing it to me.

"Thank you very much," I said and placed it in my pocketbook. "That new prescription is going to be a lifesaver for me."

Upon completion of the treatment, Rah and I went to Exam room #4. I got undressed and sat on the table. I wasn't nervous today. I felt so much better physically at that moment that even the thought of an exam was not going to spoil the fact that I was finally feeling better.

Dr. Johnson came into the room with his usual serious looking expression. "Did you receive the prescription that I wrote for your nausea?" he asked.

"Yes I did Doctor, thank you," I replied.

"Well, let's proceed with the exam,"he said sternly. I want to take a look at this tumor. Dr Merrick has sent me some excellent reports regarding your progress. I want to see the progress myself." My feet went into the stirrups, and the exam was over in a ten seconds. I can verify what Dr Merrick has observed, he stated. Definite progress has been made, he said without changing his expression. I will examine you again in about three weeks. Good bye Ms. Ayer." and he was gone in a flash.

"Mr. Personality don't you think Rah?" I asked.

"Definitely Mom, but I hear he is one of the best cancer doctors in the State," Rah replied.

"Well, we had better get moving or I am going to be late for my radiation treatment this afternoon," I said while staring to get dressed. We hurried out of the exam room and down the hall to the elevator. I was smiling. Today had turned out to be much better than I ever could have imagined.

We were in the car and driving out of the parking lot in less than five minutes and headed for the radiation treatment. My lower body was hurting so very much, it was extremely difficult for me to sit. I was so uncomfortable. The exam hadn't helped the condition at all. I was fidgeting like a child in a soiled diaper. Rah glanced at me while she was driving and asked, "Are you alright?" "Just a tad uncomfortable, but I'll make it through the radiation treatment," I stated. It was to the point now, that I was so sore I couldn't sleep. Even without any underwear and the cream, it seemed like I was fighting a losing battle. My skin was burned and raw sore. I couldn't bear anything to be touching the area and sitting comfortably was almost totally impossible. I said a prayer to the Lord at that very moment while we were driving. "Help me God, please give me the strength to with stand the coming months. But I did not forget to thank him for the good news regarding my tumor. I know that God is with me and with his guidance, I will find the strength inside me to get through all that I have in front of me.

The radiation treatment schedule was running a little behind schedule today. Apparently I was not the only one who was late. I went to my locker and changed into the dressing gown and sat in the Patients lounge and spoke with two other women who were sitting and waiting for their name to be called. I had seen both of them before but I hadn't had the opportunity to speak to them. They were both older than I and seemed to be preoccupied with their reading material. I would have liked to share my good news with them regarding my tumor, but they didn't seem to be interested in talking to me. So I picked up a medical magazine and proceeded to skim through it trying to pass the time. I had not had the opportunity to go to the library as yet, but I was still determined to do so. I still had the question in my mind where did this cancer come from. A young nurse named Carol came in to retrieve me and escort me to the radiation treatment room. I smiled and said, "good bye" to the ladies as I left the room. The radiation treatment was quick and the nurses were their usual friendly selves. I told them all about Dr. Johnson statement that he conferred with Dr. Merrick regarding my tumor. They were both so sweet and happy for me.

Mary, the smaller of the two nurses smiled, "I knew that you could beat this disease."

"Sometimes we can just tell by the patient, and Pam you are one of those special patients." I thanked her for her kind words and left the room. I must have been walking funny as Mary stopped me and asked, "Is the discomfort getting worse?"

I just shook my head yes for my answer. "Are you using the cream?" she asked acting very concerned.

"All the time without fail. I replied. Is there a stronger medicine for this condition?"

Mary said, "Honestly Pam I am not sure. Why don't you call later on this afternoon when Dr. Merrick will be here and talk to him on the phone?" she suggested.

I started walking toward the door and turned around and said, "I think I might just do that."

Sue was there in the parking lot as usual. "Hi Sue," I said getting into the car.

"Hi."

"You look exhausted Pam. Did you get any rest over the long weekend at Rah's house?" she asked.

"Sue, I practically slept the entire three day weekend, I confessed. The trouble was I was vomiting all the time, so I was really feeling lousy."

"Oh not, has that started again?" she said so concerned.

"Yes, but I have a new prescription if you wouldn't mind dropping it off at the pharmacy, it might help me."

"Of course, we will go there first and then I will bring you home. Can you make it alright? Your not feeling nauseated right now are you?"

"No right now would be fine Sue. I can make it, lets go right now as I really need the medicine as fast as I can get it," I admitted.

She immediately started the car up and headed for the pharmacy. She started to get out of the car but turned and asked, "Do you need anything else?"

"Maybe some soda, but that's it." I replied sleepily.

"I'll be right back," she said and she was gone. I sat in the car trying to find a position where I could sit and be comfortable while she was gone. I ended up getting out of the car and holding on to the door handle waiting for her. She came out with a frown on her face. "They don't have the medicine, but they are calling other pharmacies and will call me as soon as they locate the pills."

"Okay, lets go home then, I am so sleepy and I have to get out of these clothes."

We arrived back home in five minutes (it seemed like five hours, I was hurting so). I started to walk up the stairs when Sue suggested that I go to my bedroom and lie down for a while rather than climb stairs. I agreed with her and walked into my almost living room. I stepped into the room and saw the most beautiful emerald green carpet on the floor. In the kitchen was a beautiful tile floor and brand new kitchen cabinets and a kitchen sink.

"Go into the bathroom, Pam," Sue suggested. See what your son has done." I walked slowly to the bathroom door and opened it. There it was, beautiful tiled walls and tile floors. It was done in white tiles with small black diamonds set in each tile. I was stunned. "Do you like everything?" Sue asked. Brandon worked the entire three days and nights to finish it for you. Do you like the kitchen?"Sue asked. She was so excited, she actually made me laugh.

"Sue it is absolutely gorgeous. I love it. Where is Brandon now?" I asked.

"He should be back shortly, his worked called him and he had to go in for a few hours." Sue asked once again, "You really like it?"

I smiled and gave her a hug, "I think it is beautiful and I love it."

"Good, now you go rest, and when Brandon comes home I will send him down to see you." Sue stated. She gave me one more hug and returned upstairs.

I stood there in the hallway looking at the bathroom and the finished kitchen. It truly was beautiful. I walked into the living room and bent down to feel the carpet. The color was so pretty and the carpet was so soft I sat down and swept my hands back and forth feeling the texture. My eyes were so heavy and I felt so tired, I thought that I would just lie down for a minute or two and then go into my bed. I must of fallen asleep laying right in the middle of the floor.

The next thing I heard was Brandon's voice, "Mom!" "Are you okay?"

I sat up quickly and saw Brandon on the floor next to me. "Oh Bran, it's beautiful," I said and I started to cry.

"You scared me to death," he said scolding me.

"I am so sorry, I was just feeling the carpet when I must have fallen asleep," I said sheepishly.

"Well as long as you like it, now you are going to bed."

"I'll talk to you later on," and he guided me into my room and helped me onto my bed. Bran closed the bedroom door and I lay there for a few minutes thinking about my new beautiful home. What a magnificent job my son had done, and how hard he must have worked. I needed to take another moment and thank God again for everything he had given me, especially my wonderful children. Where would I be and who would I be without them.

Chapter 49

Holiday Shopping

Time was passing very rapidly and the treatments continued daily. Christmas was approaching much to my dismay. I so wanted to be able to go Christmas shopping, but there was no money coming in. The fact was I was totally broke. If someone had asked me for one dollar, I couldn't have scraped it up from the bottom of my pocketbook. I had received a few Christmas cards from some of my fellow postal workers, but no visitors. I think that they felt uncomfortable in facing me. It was for the best, I think. I still looked so thin and drawn. My vanity prevented me from calling anyone and asking them to come and visit me. But I was lonely. I had always been so busy when I was working. I thought that I had a lot of friends, but when it comes right down to who really cares about you, all you truly have is family.

This entire illness has been a slow process for me in many ways. I had never really ever been ill before. I just took my health for granted, along with everything else in life. My work had become my world after the children had moved out. My marriage was over and my faith in men had been totally shattered. I put everything I had into my kids and my marriage, and now both my children and marriage had gone their separate ways. All I had remaining was my job. Now that is even gone. Scarlett, you were one smart woman with your attitude... Tomorrow, I will think about it tomorrow.

I had gained two pounds on the last weight check in the doctors office. I now weigh 109 pounds. Slow but steady. The nurses tease me unmercifully about how tiny I am, but they mean no harm. We just make a joke out of it. The radiation building has become my second home. Even Dr. Merrick has become a friend. Yesterday I had the opportunity to wear my smiley faced boxer shorts which have been stored in my dresser drawer. I was informed that I would receive an exam by Dr. Merrick on Wednesday (the following day). I said nothing to the nurses regarding my little surprise. I wanted to tell them, but I was afraid that one of them would slip and give my little surprise away. I dressed in my regular dressing gown and received my radiation treatment. I walked to the exam room and pulled out the boxer shorts from my pocketbook and slipped into them. I covered myself with the dressing gown and waited very patiently for the doctor to arrive. I was having a difficult time not to laugh, but I managed to keep a straight face.

I was relaxing on the exam table, still fighting off the giggles, when Dr. Merrick walked into the room. "Good afternoon Ms Ayer, and how are you doing today?"

"About the usual except for the pain. That is gone, thank God," I said.

He smiled and replied, "That is why I wanted to check you today." I positioned my self normally on the table and made sure the gown was covering the boxer shorts. Dr. Merrick walked over to the sink and put on the rubber gloves and the glasses. "I believe that the exam should be less and less discomfort for you, but please tell me right away if you feel any pain," he said as he reached for the little stool.

"Oh, don't worry about that, I will let you know right away if you are hurting me."

He sat in front of me with my feet in the stirrups, but the gown was covering me up. He reached to raise the gown and place it in the proper position for the examination when he saw the smiley boxer shorts. His facial expression was absolutely priceless. He gave me the biggest surprised looked and the widest grin I had ever seen on his face in all these months of treatments. All he could say was, I am speechless, Ms Ayer. Those are the most interesting shorts I have ever seen on a patient, and that is no exaggeration. You certainly have a wonderful sense of humor," he said still smiling.

"Why thank you doctor."

"I thought you might get a kick out of them," I teased. "I know that I should behave myself, as this is serious business, but sometimes the kid comes out in me. But I will be good and remove them now."

Dr. Merrick got off the stool and turned the other way, and I removed the shorts. "Now lets get down to seeing what that tumor is doing," he remarked as the real examination began. "The tumor is shrinking nicely. I am very pleased with what is happening to it," he said. That is it for today." He looked at me and smiled again. "I shall remember this day with a smile, Ms. Ayer." He walked over to the sink and removed his gloves and washed his hands. I got up off the table and began to get dressed.

"How many more chemo treatments are you scheduled for?" he asked.

"I believe until the end of January, approximately five more weeks," I said with a big smile.

Dr Merrick then became serious, "I received some papers from Social Security and have filled them out and forwarded them to Dr. Johnson. You should be hearing regarding a decision in about a month or two as they are very slow. I feel that you should be approved without any difficult, but if you have any problems please let me know, he said with a straight face. Now you have a nice day, and don't overdue as I know that you are very fragile." He looked at me just before he opened the door, smiled and shook his head and disappeared out the door.

Sue picked me up as usual only this time the car was filled with Christmas presents. She had just left the mall. Judging from all the presents, she had been shopping for a serious amount of time and had spent a lot of money. "I bought you something that I think you will really like," she admitted. "What, tell me Sue," I said anxiously.

"It's nothing big, but I know you will appreciate the thought. Can you reach over and get the Sears bag on the back seat?"she asked.

"Sure," and I leaned over the seat and picked out the Sears bag and pulled it into the front seat with me.

"Open it," Sue said.

When I opened the bag, I had to smile. It was a little fully decorated Christmas tree for my apartment. "Thank you Sue. It would not have been a proper Christmas for me without a tree. I love it!" That little tree pleased me so there were no words that could express my feelings. I could hardly wait to get home and find just the proper place to set it up. I had always loved decorating a house for the holidays. I usually shopped until I dropped making sure that everyone got just the right present and that no one was over overlooked. My biggest joy came from watching the children open their presents. As a child my Mom had always tried her best to give my brother and I a nice Christmas with presents, but the money was slim. Most of my presents were hand made by my Uncle Eddy. I can remember one Christmas morning in particular. Uncle Eddy (Santa) had made me a me a spectacular doll house and all the little furniture that went inside. Plus I had received my first real doll.

She was called a "Tiny Tears Doll" and she cried real tears when you gave her a bottle full of water and then squeezed her gently. How I loved that doll. It's funny the things you remember. I couldn't have been more than six years old. But I can remember that doll just like it was yesterday.

Sue carried her Christmas purchases downstairs, and we decided that the best hiding place was my clothes closet. The kids would never suspect that there would be any presents hidden in there. She proudly showed me all her purchases for the girls. Sue and Bran had always made sure that their girls had wonderful Christmas's. Ra and Greg were exactly the same way. They usually had to max out their credit cards because of having four children to buy for. But they always seemed to manage.

Their house on Christmas morning looked like a toy store. We had placed the presents neatly in the rear of my clothes closet when Sue said "Pam, I have a confession to make. I hope that you will not be angry with Bran and me. We meant well."

I looked at her with a questionable look and said, "Sue you can tell me anything."

Sue sat down on my bed and motioned for me to sit next to her. Brandon and I went to see your ex." My face must have reflected my feelings as Sue quickly said, it was a big mistake. I thought that he might have changed a little and had developed a heart, but I was wrong. We explained to him that you were really suffering not only in your health condition but financially." I got upset when he suggested that you should go to welfare. My anger began to show and I told him, Well she gave you forty thousand dollars, and she never got a dime for her house because of what you had done." He promptly showed Brandon and I the door and told us to get out. Brandon's reaction was one of total disgust. He told his father, "Don't ever call me again, I want nothing more to do with you."

"Pam, I am so sorry. We meant well, and I never believed that he could be that cruel. Please don't be angry with us."

I leaned over and gave her a hug and said, "Sue don't concern yourself about my ex. He is not well. I have know that for years and I expect nothing from him. Unfortunately I am sure that it hurt Brandon very much to hear and see how mean and hateful his own father is. I am only sorry that he had to see that, and as for me, I don't need him for anything. I have gotten this far without his help, and I intend to go the distance and come out a winner. God is watching over me, and I have to keep my heart free from vengeance and try to keep forgiveness in my soul and my thoughts. So lets not concern ourselves with my ex any more. Let's put today's meeting with him in the past." I hugged her again and she gave me a smile and a sigh.

I changed the subject and said "Tomorrow I would like to try and go to the mall. Even if I just sit and look around at all the beautiful Christmas decorations and hear the holiday music playing. I feel that it is necessary to find my Christmas spirit. It will do me a world of good to remember what Christmas is all about, but I think I need to see the shoppers and the children. I can talk to God and pray for strength while enjoying all the activity going on around me."

"If that is what you want, in the meantime, are you hungry, Pam?"

"Yes, I am. What do you have good to eat?" I asked smiling. Let's go upstairs and dig up

something good and fattening," I said laughing.

"I think I can find something in that category in the refrigerator," Sue replied. We both started laughing and started walking toward the stairway to the upstairs in search of food.

While Sue and I were sitting and eating, I told Sue about my little trick on Dr. Merrick. She laughed and laughed. "Only you Pam. I bet he will never forget you," she said in between giggles. I gave her the good news regarding the shrinkage of my tumor. I told her that the pain was lessening every day, and I was requiring less and less pain medication. Things were beginning to look up. God was answering my prayers.

Later that evening Rah called. She and Sue had apparently worked out my Christmas schedule. I was informed that I would spend Christmas evening with Brandon, Sue and the girls. Then I was to be transported to Rah's house to spend Christmas morning with their family. It all sounded wonderful to me. Christmas afternoon was going to be spent with my Mom, Dad, Jay, Ann and Cheyenne. Christmas dinner was being prepared at my Mom's. It sounded like it was going to be a wonderful Christmas holiday. The only thing that was upsetting me, was the fact that I could not afford to purchase any presents. I had mulled it over and over in my mind, but I had nothing left to sell to raise money. I would have to sit and watch Christmas eve and Christmas morning without giving anyone one present that I had purchased. *I cannot find the words to express my sorrow and shame for my inability to give.*

The following morning Sue took me to radiation, and she sat and waited in the reception area for me. We were going to attempt the trip to the mall . Sue was very leery regarding taking me there, but I insisted. I had tried my best to spruce up in appearance so that I would not stand out as a skeleton in the mall. I didn't want to scare the children or any of the shoppers. I just had to attempt to get into the spirit of Christmas. The mall was the only place, other than church that would help me find Christmas.

I walked with Sue into the first store, and I was feeling pretty confident. But by the time Sue had made three purchases I was already woozy.

"Sue, I need to find a place to sit down," I confessed.

"I know right where you can sit," she replied. She guided me to the ladies fitting room and there was a chair placed right by the door. She explained to the fitting room attendant my situation, and I was given permission to sit there for as long as I needed. "Do you need to go home?" Sue asked. "Absolutely not. When you are through in this store, I can sit out in the midway and watch the shoppers, and you can finish up any more shopping that you have to do. I will be fine," I insisted. Once Sue was finished with her purchases, we made our way through the crowds to the center of the mall. I found a nice bench in the vicinity near Santa's Workshop.

"I want to sit here Sue," I said.

"I will go and get you a coffee and a doughnut. You need to get some food inside you," Sue stated. "I'll be fine. I just need to rest. This is the best seat to see everything that is going on, I especially love to watch the children. You go and do whatever you have to do. I'll be seated right here when you are finished." I sat there admiring the view. Studying the peoples faces. Listening to the little children giggle, or scream that they had to have some new toy. Most of the people looked serious and were in full concentration of what they had to accomplish. I smiled remembering what it was like taking my children with me and trying to shop. Even just grocery shopping could be a huge challenge. But I do remember my children were well behaved. Brandon being the youngest would sit in the seat of the shopping cart. Jay would sit inside of the cart itself, and Rah would hold on and assist me in steering the cart up and down the aisles. At the time it seemed like a chore and difficult to control, but not now. I would love the opportunity to relive just one moment of a shopping trip when they were only little. I would say to my grandmother some nights after putting my children to bed, "Oh I will be so glad when they are all grown up."

She would smile and then offer a piece of her wise wisdom. "Appreciate the fact you know exactly where your children are and that they are safe. When they are grown and away from you, you will always wonder if they are okay." She was exactly one hundred percent correct as usual.

The mall was decorated beautifully. The gold and silver garland were strung from the rafters and the huge Christmas ornaments were beautifully hand painted with lovely designs painted on them. The Christmas music was playing loudly with the old holiday favorites. God I loved this time of year. The huge Christmas tree was right on the other side of where I was sitting. It almost touched the ceiling. Whomever had decorated it was very creative. It was adorned with old fashioned ornaments. All the pieces were carved in wood very precisely to resemble articles of yesteryear. Items such as sleighs, sleds, rocking horses, etc. I was enjoying my self.

I studied the shoppers playing the game I use to as a child. I would try and become that person and imagine what kind of life they lived. What kind of a house they lived in, how many children did they have, and especially if they were a happy family. Did they have a Mom and a Dad. I would usually pick out one woman that I wanted to look like and dress like when I grew up. Silly little game, but it would keep me preoccupied for long periods of time. Where I was sitting, I had the ideal vantage point for playing my game. I could pick from hundreds of different faces that were walking in front of me. The time passed quickly and before I knew it Sue was standing in front of me. "Are you all through with your shopping?" I asked.

"Yes, all finished, are you ready to go home now?"

"Yes, I am Sue, and thank you for bringing me here today." I stood up and we started walking slowly through the crowds to the car.

"Did you enjoy yourself?" Sue asked. "Oh yes."

"It's the season," I said smiling.

Chapter 50
Thoughts of Gram

As this holiday approaches, my mind has been recalling memories of the Christmas's which have passed. My Grandmother has been visiting me in my dreams the last few days, which is very unusual. Although she is often in my thoughts, I seldom dream of her. Still, the memory of her is very *vivid*. My son Jason was her favorite of all her grandchildren, and I believe the last count of the number of her grandchildren was over fifty. God how she loved him. When I close my eyes, I still can see her smiling face looking at me and holding Jason in her arms. Jay could never do any wrong in her eyes. She favored him so, and I never understood exactly why. Perhaps he reminded her of one of her own children or I like to think he reminded her of me when I was a little. But everyone in the family knew that Jay was Gramma's pet.

Through the years, Gramma and I had many long conversations in the early morning hours when neither one of us could sleep. We would talk about everything. It was Gramma who told me the facts of life. It was Gramma who tried to explain what true love felt like. I could ask her anything. It was she who told me I was pregnant before I even knew it myself. She said, "you have the glow." Gramma was always right, and she was always there for me when I needed her.

When I was a child, Gramma loved Christmas, and would celebrate it with all her heart and soul. She was always shopping and wrapping presents or writing Christmas cards or humming Christmas carols. The Christmas spirit was truly living in her. Then one Christmas eve when I was about 10 years old, my Uncle Rob who was her oldest son (he was about 45 at the time) committed suicide. I can recall Gramma talking about how very despondent he had become was when his wife had left. His wife had suddenly packed up one day and disappeared with another man, leaving him to raise their six young boys. Gramma had been staying with him that holiday to help him care for the children. Apparently Uncle Rob arose in the middle of the night on Christmas eve and decided life was not worth living. He connected a hose coming from the muffler of the car, inserting it into the inside of the car and quietly waited for the fumes to consume him. It was Gramma who found him that morning, and she could never celebrate Christmas the same ever again. She used to talked to me about her feelings years later. I can't imagine the pain she suffered. I know he left no note or explanation as to the reason for the suicide, but Gramma always blamed her self for not staying awake that night and watching him. I would sit next to her and put my arms around her when she would cry as she talked about her son.

Gram passed away when she was ninety two years old. Our last conversation together was the day before she died. We talked about how tired she was of living and the pain of out living three of her four children was more than she could bear. My mom was her only remaining child. Her youngest son, my Uncle Eddy, died the year before from Lou Gehrig disease, and her daughter, my Aunt Grace, had died this year of a heart attack. I remember her last words that she spoke to me, "Pam, I am so tired, and I don't want you to cry when I die."

"It's time to let me go and join my children." She made me promise that I would not wish her back. She talked softly while she laid in her bed in the nursing home. "I've lived a long a full life, and I have no regrets."

"But now it's time for me to return to God and my children."

"I want you to be happy for me that I will finally be in peace." I held her hand and gave her my promise. She instructed me on all her desires regarding her funeral. The last smile that she gave me was caused by her remark regarding her hair. She may have been ninety two years old, but she was still a woman. She was depending on me to make sure that her hair looked beautiful at her funeral.

The doctor said that Gram died in her sleep, and she died very peacefully. The strangest thing about her death was I was actually in the parking lot of the nursing home that night. Something unexplainable kept me from visiting her. I forced my ex to turn the car around, and we returned home. I could not force myself to go in that building to see her. That very night, the phone awakened me from my sleep around midnight. Gram had passed away. It upset me to the point that I was hysterical to think that I had not had the chance to say good bye. I was heartsick. There were so many things I wanted to say to her and ask her. But I realized now it had been God's plan for me not to be with her that night.

I followed her instructions regarding her funeral to the letter. I sat in the funeral home with the entire family, and I never shed a tear. Everything was done exactly the way she had requested. I handled the funeral myself, picking out the casket, her clothes and made sure her hair looked extra ordinally beautiful. I always did as I was told. I still miss her every day of my life. Without her guidance and strength, I would not be the woman I am today.

Every day as I drove to work, I passed the cemetery where she is buried. For the life of me I cannot make myself stop and visit her grave. I have only been to her grave on special occasions, such as her birthday, Memorial day, or Mother's day. I cannot contain my tears if I go there, and I know that is not what she wanted me to do. So I think about her with a smile and a lump in my throat.

Now, because of all these thoughts of Gramma, it's time for me to visit the shower.

Chapter 51

Christmas Eve and Christmas Day

I sat watching Alex and Bri open all their Christmas presents. The way they ripped through the wrapping paper reminded me of little tornados. Little Bri received her usual new Barbie doll and about ten new stunning outfits for the doll. Plus lots of books on archeology. Bri was very serious about becoming an archeologist when she was "all grown up" as she put it. She never wavered when I asked her what she wanted to be. The answer was always the same, an archeologist. I believe very strongly that is exactly what she will be as an adult. She has plans to go to college and study very hard.

Now Alex, that's something of a different story. Alex received mostly pretty clothes and play make-up and jewelry. Alex has different desires regarding her future. She wants children. She wants to get married and have lots of children. I have tried to talk to her, but she is very set in her ways, and really doesn't want to listen to my advise about going to college. So, I just leave it alone and keep my fingers crossed that she will change her attitude later on in life.

Brandon and Sue gave me a lovely white bathrobe as my Christmas gift. I had to laugh even though I was upset that they had gone ahead and purchased a gift for me. Brandon had this running joke about my ugly green bathrobe that I wore all the time. If I were to be honest, I would say he was absolutely correct in his description of my green robe. I wore it because it was warm and comfortable. Being so thin, I was always cold no matter what the temperature was set on. I would have the ugly green robe on over my clothes usually when Brandon came home from work. He would come down stairs to check up on me and see me sitting there wearing it. He would automatically crack a few jokes regarding my appearance and then give me his award winning smile.

The lump in my throat eased with the type of present the robe represented. It was kind of a gentle joke. Sue and Bran both knew that I did not want them to purchase a gift for me for Christmas. I had asked everyone to skip over me and concentrate only on the children and their mates. I could not give them anything, therefore it would have made it easier for me if they did not give me a present. Next year when Christmas comes, I will be physically better and perhaps things will have improved financially for me. I will make up my lack of ability to buy for anyone next year.

The door bell rang, and it was Rah, Tawnee, and Haley. Time to get my little suitcase again. Haley and Tawnee were a little confused by Alex and Brianna's ability to get their presents on Christmas Eve. Haley asked me, "Did Santa already come here?" I just shook my head yes and gave her the signal of don't say anything more! Sue did not believe in letting her children believe in Santa when they reached the age six or seven. "They are old enough to know the truth. I want them to realize that it's Mommy and Daddy who buy all the presents," she would say defiantly. Therefore the agreement was made with Alex and Bri not to discuss their disbelief in Santa with any other children.

In that way, another child's belief could not be spoiled. Sue's opinion regarding Santa did bother me though. I can't see the harm in letting a little child believe in Santa Claus. But I kept my opinion to myself and stayed away from the subject. Rah's children were taught the total opposite. Tawnee was nine and still believed in Santa. I don't believe she had ever questioned the reality of Santa. Haley and Kyle (name) were years younger, so I know there was no doubt in their young minds. They could hardly wait to get home and go to bed so that Santa would visit their home.

The children were in the bedroom enjoying the new presents while we stayed in the living room enjoying Christmas eve with laughter and egg nog. My discomfort was under control, the new prescription was working and I was wearing boxer shorts. I am sure Dr. Merrick would be proud of me. I have to admit that he was correct. If I had to wear underwear, the boxer shorts were the most comfortable for my problem. We talked for a while and then it was time to leave for Ra's house. It was getting late and Ra still had presents she needed to wrap. I wished Bran and Sue a Merry Christmas, and I kissed the girls goodbye. I was on my way to a new Christmas celebration at my daughters house. If the truth was known, I would have loved to have just gone to bed. I was so tired and was not looking forward to sleeping on a couch. But I wanted to see Rah's children have Christmas morning and that meant some discomfort on my part. So once again I was on the road traveling.

The drive to Rah's house with the children was filled with excitement an the usual threats of "you had better go to sleep when we get home or Santa won't come." How many times have I said that statement myself? I smiled remembering my children on Christmas eve. I think they must have gotten in and out of bed twenty times before they finally went to sleep. I tried to calm the kids down a little in the car by telling them to watch in the sky for Santa's sleigh. It was a very cold night and the stars were very bright. It did side track them for a short while. They spotted an airplane in the sky and Haley was sure it had to be Santa. I assured her she was probably correct. Rah and I just smiled and didn't say a word, while the children whispered to each other and giggled the rest of the ride home.

When we arrived at Rah's, the children jumped out of the car and ran into the house. "They'll have their pajamas on by the time we get in the door," Rah commented. "Yes your right, then it will take another hour or so before they actually fall asleep their so excited."

"You and your brothers were just like that when it came to Christmas."

Rah had decorated her home beautifully. Their Christmas tree was huge. How Rah and Greg even got it into the living room, I will never know. Each year their tree got bigger and bigger. I believe that Rah and Brandon had some kind of contest going on as to who could get the biggest tree. I went immediately to the couch and sat down. The kids came out of their bedrooms dressed in their pajamas and were ready to go to bed. I told them that I would watch for Santa, and that if I should wake up when he came in, I would tell him how well behaved they have been all year. Smiles and kisses were given to all, and they were off to bed.

Rah had the usual last minute wrapping of presents to do but she had to wait and make sure the children were asleep. She gave me a glass of wine and we sat and talked about the Christmas she and her brothers shared. "Mom, you sure made our Christmas's special, "she said smiling.

"We had some great ones didn't we?"

"Yes we did."

"Enjoy this time with your children Rah, as the years fly by and Christmas is no fun without children."

It was around 11:00 p.m. when Rah and Greg began bringing out the presents and placing them under the tree. Rah spread out the remaining presents that had to be wrapped on the living room floor (just as I used to do) and around twelve midnight everything was set for the early morning chaos to begin. After Greg and Rah said their good night they retired to their bedroom, both of them looking exhausted. I sat and watched the usual Christmas movie, "It's a wonderful life" and eventually fell asleep.

Somewhere around three a.m. I was awakened by someone standing next to me near the couch. It was little Tawnee. "What's the matter little one?"

"I had to go to the bathroom Meme," she said sleepily.

I got up and walked her carefully and quietly to the bathroom and then back to her little bed. Haley was still sound asleep. I tucked little Tawnee into her bed and kissed her softly. I think she was back to sleep in seconds. Now I was wide awake, so I made myself a pot of coffee and turned on the lights of the Christmas tree. I stared at the tree with all the presents underneath it and gave thanks to God for letting me be alive to share in this moment. I prayed for forgiveness regarding my pride for not being able to purchase any gifts for my family. The only gift I can give them is in my heart and that is my love for all of them. I fell back to sleep talking to God.

Six o'clock arrived and so did the children. Like gang busters out of their bedrooms. Mass confusion occurring almost immediately. Greg was the official organizer. He calmed the children down and handed out the presents in an orderly fashion. I sat and watched the entire scene of the unwrapping of all the presents. What a joy it is to watch little children on Christmas morning. Their faces glow with happiness and surprise. I was so fortunate to have such a beautiful family. It's the best present any mother could ask for. I was surrounded by happiness.

Ms. Amanda came shuffling out from her bedroom at this point. Her nausea problems had ceased and she was beginning to get a little chubby in the tummy area. I looked at her and I suddenly realized that I was soon to be a great grandmother. I prayed to God at the very moment to take care of Amanda and the child she was carrying. I just could not imagine Amanda being a mother. She was a child herself looking for her Christmas presents from Santa. My heart sank into my chest. "Give me strength," I thought.

Rah had purchased some very pretty new clothes that Amanda could wear without anyone being able to know she was pregnant. I know that it was difficult for Amanda in school being so young, and being talked about. Sometimes children can be very mean. But Amanda was tough, and was determined not to let anything bother her. She carried on each day as if there was nothing unusual going on in her life.

"Hi Meme, Merry Christmas!" Amanda said when she noticed me sitting there.

"Merry Christmas to you Ms. Amanda."

"I don't have the chance to see you very often. How have you been feeling?"

Amanda smiled, "I have been feeling great. The doctor says I am doing fine and so is the baby."

"Meme, do you think I will have a little girl?" she asked. "Amanda, I have told you before that I would have to guess and say no. I think the baby your carrying is a little boy. Sorry, I know that you want a little girl, but I have never been wrong. You might want to plan on buying only blue outfits."

A disappointed look crossed her face and she asked again, " Any chance at all you might be wrong?"

"Sorry little girl, but I feel very strongly he is a definitely a boy."

Rah got into the conversation, "You had better listen to Meme, if she says it's a boy, it's a boy."

Rah got herself out of the chair and walked over to me carrying a small package. She gave me her little girl smile and said, "Open it Mom."

My hands started to tremble as I opened the small package very carefully. Inside was a beautiful gold bracelet decorated with small diamonds and garnets. "How could you afford something like this?" "Don't ask questions, Mom. Do you like it?"

I was so emotional the words were having trouble getting out of my mouth. I didn't want to cry, but it was unavoidable. "It's beautiful," I stated while crying my eyes out. "Help me put it on Rah."

She snapped the clasp and gave me a kiss and a hug. "Merry Christmas Mom."

Just then a voice yelled from the kitchen. "Is anyone hungry?"

"Yes I am," I answered. "Well, I am going to start cooking right now." Greg said. "Breakfast should be ready in about a half an hour." I sat there watching the kids enjoy all the new presents. Santa had brought them some new games for the Nintendo machine, new dolls, toy guns and trucks. Rah's living room looked like a toy store. I was really feeling very sleepy and tired. I hadn't really fallen back to sleep since Tawnee had awaken me. I wasn't in any pain, and my stomach wasn't bothering me. I was just tired and very uncomfortable. My day was just beginning. The next stop was my Mom's house for Christmas

249

dinner with my parents and Jay and Ann.

Greg prepared a wonderful Christmas breakfast. Eggs, bacon, ham, toast, home fries and coffee. I was starving and didn't have a problem eating everything on my plate. Greg was definitely a great cook. By the time everyone was finished there was nothing left of the table to even nibble on. It seemed that everyone enjoyed Greg's cooking. After breakfast I excused myself and went into Amanda's room to see if I could catch on my sleep. I slept for a couple of hours when Amanda came in to tell me it was almost time for me to go to my Mom's. The nap helped me quite a bit and I was feeling quite a bit better. I got up and headed for the shower to make myself presentable for the rest of the family. The children were still in the living room playing with all the new toys, laughing and yelling as I walked through the room. Christmas had definitely arrived.

Dad and Mom arrived about an hour later to pick me up. They came in with their bags of presents for the kids. Rah gave her presents to my parents and we shared some more coffee and conversation. Needless to say, there was more excitement and wrappings for Rah to pick up when the exchange of gifts was over with. I smiled as I looked at her. I knew she was exhausted and the day was far from over. She would be having company all day long. Many more family members would be visiting with more presents and more wrapping paper to be picked up off the floor. It was going to be a long day for her and all the other mothers of the world.

When my parents and I arrived back to their apartment, all you could smell was food cooking. Mom had prepared a wonderful dinner and was very cheerful. Within ten minutes of our arrival home, the doorbell rang and Jay and his family were standing at the door. Presents were again passed out while little Cheyenne slept in her carrier which was placed carefully on the floor next to the Christmas tree. She was dressed in a green velvet outfit and resembled a child's Christmas doll.

Jay explained how work had been slow because of the winter weather. He and Ann were struggling with their finances right now. Ann was unable to work because of the baby, and Jay's line of seasonal work made it extremely difficult for them to manage. I used to be able to assist them with money when I was working but unfortunately my hands were tied right now. Jay said that he had signed up for unemployment last week, but hadn't heard anything regarding an approval or denial for his benefits as yet.

Ann asked, "How do you like living at Brandon's and Sue's, Pam?"

It's good, they are great to me and the location is very convenient for my radiation treatments. It has work out very well so far. Brandon has worked very diligently on my apartment, and it was practically completed. So I have no complaints," I confessed smiling. Jay had gone into the kitchen and was sampling some of the food when Ann explained that Jay had been arguing with his father. Apparently, my ex had called Jay and the conversation got a little out of hand regarding me. My ex had given Jay the same cold reaction about me and Jay did not like it. Harsh words were spoken and any plans to visit Jays father today were put on hold. My ex, it seems, will be spending Christmas day without seeing any of his children or grandchildren.

My Mom called everyone into the kitchen to enjoy her Christmas dinner. It was a typical New England dinner. Ham, sweet potatoes, squash, etc. Everything was there except for Gramma's Christmas pudding. Gramma was the only person who knew how to prepare it and she had taken the receipt with her when she died. The only thing I can remember about her pudding is that she prepared it and placed it in a coffee can. Then it was baked in the over.

The phone rang twice during dinner. The first call was from Brandon. He wished everyone a Merry Christmas, and then spoke with Jay for a few minutes making arrangements to meet him at Rah's house for their exchange of gifts. The second call was from my brother Edward. He sounded as jolly as Santa Clause. I spoke with him for a few minutes and then turned the phone over to Mom. My mother beamed as she talked with him. Edward could still do no wrong in her eyes, and I was very glad that he had remembered to call. He told Mom he was presently living in Texas and would remain there until spring. After that he wasn't sure where he and Fern would be going. Mom gave me back the phone and Edward and I talked for a few minutes.

"You have a wonderful Christmas Pam, and take care of yourself," he said.

"I will," I promised. You and Fern enjoy your Christmas." We spoke a minute or two longer and said good bye. The lump in my throat was making an appearance. I miss him more now then I ever have. I am ashamed of myself for taking my brother's love for granted the way I have over all these years. But I am thankful to God that I was given the opportunity to realize how much I love him before it was too late.

Ann and Jay said their farewell after dinner and were on the way to Rah's house. It had been a very long day, and I needed to rest. I was so full from Greg's breakfast and Mom's dinner, I thought I was going to explode. All I wanted to do at this moment was go to sleep. I remember hearing Mom in the kitchen, and seeing Dad in his recliner watching a football game and thinking Merry Christmas to all.

Chapter 52
New Years

I slept the rest of the evening and into the early morning hours on my mom's couch. I was still feeling exhausted. Today I am not going anywhere. I am not even going to get dressed, I thought. I was feeling as if I had been hit by a truck, and every bone in my body was aching. All I wanted to do today was relax. As much as I loved my family, I did not feel the need to entertain any company. Just me and television set, no phone, and no visitors. I can deal with my parents as they are quite and need very little of my attention. Both my Mom and Dad usually fall asleep if they sit down in their perspective favorite chairs. Even my appetite needed a vacation. I had eaten so much food yesterday it was truly a miracle I wasn't up and vomiting all night long. I am sure that the only reason I didn't get sick is the new prescription medicine that Dr. Johnson had prescribed for me.

It was daylight, but both my parents were still sleeping. It never ceases to amaze me how they manage what they do at their age. Nothing seems to slow them down. They face problems without blinking an eye. I can't help but wonder how I will be at that age, if I make it that long. Perhaps with age does come wisdom. I have heard that saying all my life, but I never really believed it was accurate. I always thought if you were stupid when you were young, there is a good chance that you will be stupid when your old.

I hope that my parents don't mind if I stay here for the next few days. I love my children and all the grandchildren, but I am so physically exhausted I need some total down time. No kids at all. Monday will come quick enough and the treatments will resume whether I am tired or not. Things are getting more difficult for me to withstand, and the end of the chemo treatments can't come fast enough. I know that I am almost there. If all goes well, there will be only four more chemo treatments. Once I get them over with, perhaps I will begin to feel stronger. The radiation is hard, but does not drain the life out of me. I just have to hold on a little longer.

As always, Dad was the first one up and moving about. I could hear him humming as he moved around the apartment. He hums or whistles all the time. I know that he is not aware that he does whistle and hum. If I were to ever question him about it, I am sure that he wouldn't have the slightest idea what I was talking about. Strange, but I have always found the sound of his humming very comforting and soothing. As a child, when Dad was humming I knew that everything was fine and my world was safe place. I could see him as he walked from the hallway going into the kitchen. He peeked in the living room to check up and on and saw that I was awake and smiling at him. "Oh your already awake, why don't you try and sleep a little longer Pam. It's still very early in the morning. Have you been awake very long?" he asked.

"No, Dad I just woke up a short time ago. I am still feeling tired and just want to rest and relax today. Christmas took a lot out of me. Would you and Mom mind if I stayed her for the next couple of days? I really need some quiet."

He smiled, "Of course not, you don't have to even ask. You can stay as long a you want or need to. Your mother was right again yesterday when she said that you looked exhausted. You did to much traveling, and you should have stayed in one place and just took it easy."

I smiled, "I know your right Dad, but you know how I am about Christmas. Christmas wouldn't be the same if there were no children around me. I couldn't bear the fact of spending Christmas alone no matter how sick I was feeling. Just being surrounded by my family made my Christmas special. I wouldn't want to have been my ex husband yesterday. I know that none of the children even called him yesterday. As crazy as it sounds Dad, I actually feel sorry for him."

Dad looked at me a little puzzled and said, "You know that I have never been one to say anything bad about anyone, but your ex has a severe problem. He should have never done those things to you regarding the house. He knew that what he had done was going to cause a major problem when it came to selling the house. That is the reason that he gave it up to you without some sort of fight. "I know Dad, but lets not start our day by talking about him. I have too much to be thankful for, and I know that things are only going to get better for me as time goes by."

We changed the subject and went on to the discussion about breakfast. I knew that Dad would give me a little problem about not eating.

"I am really not hungry. Just fix something for yourself and Mom. I will eat a little later on. I just want to lay here and try and go back to sleep for a little while, if you don't mind?"

"Okay, you rest and I will try and be as quiet as possible. But when your mother gets up, I want you to go into our bedroom where you can have some privacy." I smiled and said, "that's a deal."

The rest of my day was spent in and out of sleep. I heard the phone ring occasionally but Mom must of informed anyone that called I was sleeping. I'll call them back when I finally feel strong enough to walk into the living room, I thought to myself. My body kept having the sensation of drifting, and I would fall into a semi-conscious state. I was not awake, but I was not asleep. When I was conscious, my mind kept returning to the thought of dying. In the past few months I had realized there was a strong possibility that I might have to leave this earth whether I wanted to or not. Funny thing though, I wasn't even scared about it. My biggest fear was not for myself but for my children. I wished I had taken out a huge life insurance policy so that everyone would be taken care. But who really ever thinks they are going to die? My children would just have to get by on the small amount of insurance money that I had left them. At least it's something, I thought. But I must write out a will. I can't keep putting it off,…. just in case.

It wasn't until around 9:30 p.m. that I walked into the living room. My poor parents. They were accustomed to going to bed at eight o'clock every night. I apologized for keeping them from getting into their own bed.

They both asked if I was feeling better, and I told them, "Yes." I said you two just go bed, and I was feeling much stronger, (lying) and not to concern themselves about me tonight. "Just go to bed and you get some rest."

"I am planning on taking a much needed shower and then watch some television." My Mom gave me that "look" and then said, "good night."

I sat on the couch for a while until I was sure that they were asleep and then made my way to the bathroom. It had been quite a few days since I had cried, and my body was calling out to me. Let it out Pam. You'll feel better once the tears come. I had fought off any tears for the Christmas celebration. But Christmas was over and a new year was approaching fast. I opened the shower doors and stepped inside.

After my shower I felt some relief. With New Years Eve right around the corner I had to make my decision on what I wanted to do. I really did not feel up to a repeat of Christmas. I feel so very ill, and weak. I shall talk to Brandon and Rah and see if I can get them to go out and let me sit with the children. The kids are never any problem for me. I can watch them play their video games and perhaps we will rent a movie. I shall bring up that idea tomorrow when I talk to Rah.

The week passed and I continued with my treatments wearing my usual smile. Oh, I am just fine, and feeling stronger. I just wish I could just once state the truth, No, I am not good. I wish I could sit down without discomfort and eat until I burst. I cannot stand the thought of another day of radiation and chemo. I am not strong and happy. I am weak and I want to cry all the time. But that is not allowed. I have to be brave. No one likes a complainer, and I don't want to worry anyone. So I shall go on only thinking the truth, but never saying it. God forgive me.

It was decided (I am not sure who decided it) that I would spend New Years Eve home with Rah and Greg. Apparently they had a rule about not going anywhere on New Years Eve. My children were not drinkers or party goers. Greg went out and bought shrimp and champaign for the evenings celebration at home. Brandon Sue, Jay, and Ann were all staying home tonight as well. I won't have to worry that anyone of them are out on the road with all the drunk drivers. So therefore I got my wish in a way. I got to stay home with some of the children and rest knowing that my family were safe and sound at home. I didn't even stay up to see the new year make it's grand entrance. Brandon called around 9:30p.m. to wish me a Happy New Year. He had assumed that I would be sleeping at midnight so he made the decision to call me early. He was right. I fell asleep by 10:00 p.m. But before I fell asleep, I made a promise to myself that next year was going to be totally different. I would celebrate New Years Eve with all my family. I was determined to live my life with gratitude and enjoy each moment as it comes. Next year I will look back on tonight as my wake up call to begin living a different type of life. A life full of love and thankfulness. God give me the courage and strength to never forget how quickly everything you have and love can be taken away from you. My New Years resolution is to never take anything for granted again.

Chapter 53
Last Chemo

I was smiling during my morning shower. Today is going to be my last chemo treatment (if all goes well). I was so excited and I couldn't wait to get there and get it over with. When Rah walked in the living room she was smiling also. "This is it, Mom. Your almost there."

I hugged her and said, "I know, I can't believe it. Just the thought of not having that poison pumped into my veins is a wonderful thing. I can take the radiation, even with all the discomfort it causes me. But maybe now I will start feeling stronger, and not so sick all the time."

Rah gave me a big smile, "Are you ready to go?"

"Oh God yes, lets get there and get it over with."

I went for my last blood test, and happily informed the nurse that this was my final day. She smiled and said, "I am very happy for you. Good luck with the rest of your life."

When Rah and I walked into the waiting room, the room was full. There were a lot of new faces sitting that I had not seen before. I particularly noticed a young woman (somewhere in her late 30's) sitting with her mother in the very back of the room. I knew that today was her first visit. It was her facial expression and her mother's concerned look that was the major tip off. Her Mom was holding her hand trying to comfort her. I felt something so strong for her, I wanted to walk over to her and comfort her as well. But unfortunately I felt uncomfortable about doing so.

My name was called and Rah started walking ahead of me. At the very last minute I hesitated and turned and walked over to the young woman her. I stood in front of her and she looked up at me. "You'll do fine."

"I made it, and so will you." She looked at me for a second and then she smiled. Her mother looked at me and simply said, "thank you." I touched their hands with mine and continued on my way with Rah standing and waiting for me at the double doors.

All the nurses were smiling and congratulating me on this being my last treatment. I told them how much their kindness had meant to me. I really appreciated everything that they had done for me. I sat and watched as the final IV was placed in my vein. My lab test came back and the nurse was given the go ahead to proceed with the treatment. Four hours later Rah and I walked out the front door laughing and celebrating. I could hardly contain my joy. I wanted to yell to the world that I had made it through one of the worse experiences in my entire life. I kept silently saying "thank you God, thank you." I said to Rah, "next stop radiation, and then total annihilation of my tumor." I held on the Rah's hand, and said "Thank you for being here with me through all of this. I could not have made it without you."

Rah just squeezed my hand and smiled.

"I'll talk to you tomorrow Rah," I said while sliding out of the front seat. "Bye Mom."

When I walked into the radiation building, my joy must have showed all over my face. "Ms. Ayer you look wonderful," the receptionist said as I approached her.

"I just finished my chemo treatments and I couldn't be happier."

"Congratulations" she said smiling.

"I'm almost finished. I'm almost there," I added. Naturally I had to share my joy with my two radiation nurses. Sweet Mary was quick to add, "Well you only have about twelve more weeks of radiation to endure and you will be finished here as well. You have come a long way, and I must tell you that you have been the bright spot in our day. Every time you came for your treatment you brought a smile to everyone you went anywhere near. We will miss you around here."

I smiled at her and said, "thank you. You two have become my friends and my close confidants. I shall never forget you."

I asked Mary, "Do you think I will be feeling physically stronger soon? I mean without the chemo being put into me?"

"Well, the radiation treatments have their own side effects, but I do think some of your strength will return. Nausea is not a radiation side effect usually.

Especially in the area you have been receiving it."

"The only other thing I wish that I knew is where this cancer came from?" I confessed. "I have been trying to get to the library for months, but I never seem to make it there."

Mary looked at me and said, "Perhaps it would be better for you to ask Dr. Merrick that question. Medical books can be confusing to say the least. It would be to your advantage to get the information from a doctors point of view. We all know that you should have gotten your pap smears on a regular basis. The treatment would have been far less invasion and devastating. But the pap smear would not of prevent the cancer from forming. You would have had to already had the cancer for the smear to detect it. So Pam, talk to Dr Merrick during your next exam. Which by the way will be this Friday."

"Oh that is just peachy. I look forward to those exams like being shot with a gun."

Mary burst into laughter. "I can tell you this, "Your exam will be in the larger room where you received your tattoos, so you might want to prepare yourself for a very through exam."

"Ugh," was all I could say.

The treatment got underway and was over quickly. As I was sliding off the table Mary touched my hand and quietly said, "if you are determined to go to the library look under pap smear." It will be listed under Cervical Cancer. That is all I can tell you right now."

I knew from the look on her face what I was about to find out regarding my disease was in no way going to make me happy. I hurriedly got dressed and headed for the parking lot. I wanted to share my happiness with Sue regarding the end of chemo. I also wanted to ask her to take me to the library. I was hearing that little voice in the back of my mind saying, "better not go."

"Wait until you talk to the doctor." But I couldn't wait any longer. Today was the day. I had made up my mind.

I was smiling when I got into the front seat of Sue's car. "Is chemo all over with?" Sue asked.

"Yes it is. Now for a favor from you. Sue, I need you to bring me to the library. I have to look my disease up. I can't put it off any longer. Would you mind driving me there?"

"Of course I wouldn't mind. I'll have you there in five minutes." She asked me all about how my treatment went and I answered her, but my mind was somewhere else. My mind was in the library where the answer to my question was about to be answered.

Sue and I walked in the front door of the Fairfield Public Library and I was shaking like a leaf. "Why are you so upset? I thought you would be happy today."

I looked at Sue and simply said, "I am about to find out where and how I got this disease, and I know that I am not going to be very pleased with the answer."

"The nurse at radiation told me to look under Cervical Cancer, the "Human Papilloma Virus." "Does that sound like something that is going to make me smile."

"I don't think so." I walked down the main isle as if I were drawn by some sort of magnet pulling me toward the medical area. In a flash of a minute I was standing right in front of hundreds of books on Cancer. I reached for the first one my hand could touch. I checked the index for the page number of Cervical Cancer. The page flipping took only a second. I read the first three paragraphs without taking a breath. My legs became weak, the room began to spin. Sue grabbed me and directed me to a desk and a chair when I totally collapsed. HPV...Human Papilloma Virus. I handed the book to Sue and pointed to where she should read.

Did he give you this cancer?"

"I just don't know what to think any more," I said crying quietly.

She gently put her arm around me, "What can I say to comfort you?"

"Nothing, I had to find out and now I know." You see these books explains that there are three ways of contacting this virus, (1) Having intercourse at an early age. (2). Having too many sexual partners . (3) Having unprotected sex.

I sat there and calmed myself down. I tried to sort it all out in my mind. I had never had sex until I was married. I had been a virgin when I was married, so the idea of a lot of sexual partners was out of the question, but I did have unprotected sex with my husband, for the thirty some years we were married. Why wouldn't I? He was my husband God forgive me for thinking hateful thoughts. I prayed to God right there in the library, "Please give me the strength to forgive."

"I know that hatred and revenge in my heart will only make me sicker than I am already. I think at that moment I truly wanted to die. Had Sue not been with me or if I had been alone somewhere and read about this, I really might had done something terrible. But once again the good Lord was with me and protecting me. I was not alone, and I had a second chance in life. I was not going to let thoughts of him destroy me anymore. If this is true, someday he will answer for his actions to a much higher power than me.

"Okay Sue, I am ready now. Let's go home and not speak of this to anyone. I don't want anyone to know about this right now."

"I am too ashamed." I felt as if my heart had been smashed and stomped on. I wanted to go home and take a shower....I thought, *how would my hero handle this? The answer is ....tomorrow.*

Chapter 54

A Brand New Year

As each day passed, the days became more and more blurry to me . One day melted into the next. Every day was just like the last. Today was Friday I think, and I was scheduled for an exam by Dr. Merrick. How I dreaded just the thought of another exam. I was so very tired of it all. The fear that something new would be found, was always in my mind. I kept thinking, what if the cancer starts to spread? Would I be strong enough to fight it? I never dreamed that I would have to face such a disease. I kept telling myself that I was getting better. The treatments were doing what they were supposed to do. But I had that constant fear in the back of my mind all the time. What if? I knew that I had to remain in a positive frame of mind, but it was so hard sometimes.

Recently I had been thinking about retiring from my job. I didn't feel as if I could go back to work. All my friends, or at least I thought they were my friends had deserted me. No one ever even made an attempt to call me or send me a card in all these months. No, I am wrong there. My friend Joan has called a few times. But I know she is busy with her life and has enough problems of her own. I guess that is what happens in most cases. It would be so nice to talk to someone not in the family. I might be able to express how I really feel instead of trying to hide my emotions all the time. Perhaps when all this is over with I will go an see a counselor. I should be happy that my condition seems to be improving, but in truth, I am anything but happy.

As for my trip to the library, I don't believe that did my attitude any good. I have really tried to put it out of my mind, but it is extremely difficult to do. The fact is, the more I think about it the angrier I become. Every time I lie on the table and receive a radiation treatment, I think of what has caused me to be there. I am trying very hard not to ask the question, why me Lord, but it creeps into my thoughts constantly. It's time for me to stop all this thinking and get myself out of bed and face Dr Merrick.

I got up and finally got myself dressed. I am so nervous about this exam this morning. I wonder why the special exam room. What was Dr. Merrick looking for? I know I have to stop driving myself crazy with all these questions. The answer is only about forty five minutes away. I can already hear Sue and the girls moving around upstairs.

My apartment was really looking very nice. I had been given some pictures and small articles to place around the living room by some of Sue's family. The living room just needed a small couch and a chair to be complete. Sue had mentioned to me that she had noticed a nice set in a furniture store not far from her work. We are going to go there and see if they do lay-a-ways. Of course I could always rent a living room set, but how would I make the payments? I still have no money coming in. Money wasn't tight, it was invisible. But at least I wasn't starving. Sue and Brandon made sure that I ate well. I realize that I still eat like a bird, but now without chemo perhaps my appetite will be returning. I started my way to upstairs when I met Sue coming down stairs to make sure I was up and moving around. "Good morning." I said.

"Your up already?" Sue asked.

"Yes, I want to go a little early this morning and get this exam over with. I am a nervous wreck about it," I confessed.

"You'll do fine, Pam," Sue replied. Look how far you have come in the past months. Please don't make yourself sick worrying. It doesn't do you any good. Let me just tell the girls that we are leaving." she requested.

"Tell them I said I will see them later on today. I will just go and get my coat and we can be on our way," I turned around and walked back downstairs.

Sue was getting into the car when I came out the front door. Alex and Bri were standing in the picture window waving. Sue yelled to them, "I will be right back. Make sure the front door is locked." Alex yelled back, "I will mommy. Bye Meme."

I smiled and waved and sat down in the car and shut the door. "They always cheer my day. I don't know what I would do without my grandchildren. Sometimes it seems like they are all I have to keep me going and not giving up."

Sue smiled and said, "They all love you so much. You have to get better."

The parking lot was full as usual at the treatment center. I told Sue, as I was leaving the car, to come in and wait for me if I was not out at my usual time. I might be longer than usual, and I don't want you to be freezing out here in the car."

"Stop your worrying about me. If you don't come out, I will go in and wait. You just get yourself in there and do what you have to do. Good luck."

I walked in and headed straight for the locker area. I changed into my dressing gown and walked to the Patients Lounge. As I walked in I said my usual "Good morning." And as usual I got the same results. A few nods and a few mumbles. I sat in the chair by the television and began watching the program that was playing. It was about fifteen minutes before the nurse came to get me.

"Hi Pam, follow me," she said.

"Hi Mary, what the heck are they going to do to me today? Do you have any idea?"

She looked at me questionably and admitted, "No not really, but I have a suspicion that it has something to do with the brand new radiation equipment they are preparing. All I know that it some super machine and everyone is very excited about it's capabilities. I suspect that you are going to be the first candidate for its use."

"Well, that sounds like a barrel of fun," I admitted. We walked into the exam room and there were already four people standing around the table. I recognized Dr. Merrick's assistant Dr. Evens.

"Good morning Ms Ayer. We are all set up for you. Dr. Merrick will be in momentarily, please have a seat on the table."

I lay down on the table and thought, they are going to take ex-rays. That's all that this machine did the last time. Only they used that terrible white stuff. Oh brother, this is going to be fun. I hated that stuff. I had no sooner thought that when Dr. Merrick walked in.

"Good morning and how is my favorite little patient today?"

"So far I am fine," I answered. But what are you planning to do to me this morning?"

He smiled and said, "Nothing to bad, just uncomfortable for you."

"Okay, lets get this over with." My legs were put into the stirrups and draped with a white linen cloth. Then the white liquid was inserted into my rectum and into my vagina. Not a very comfortable feeling, but far from as painful as it was the first time. Dr. Merrick saw me grimace and asked how I was feeling. "Are you in pain?" he asked. I looked directly at Dr. Merrick and said, "This is the closest thing to sex that I have had in five years." Well let me tell you the expression on Dr. Merrick's face was worth my being so uncomfortable. He looked at me with such a shocked expression as if he could not believe what he just heard. I know he tried not to, but he had been taken over by the giggles. He turned and left the room saying only, "I will return in a moment." Everyone else in the room was trying with out much success to conceal their smiles. I just laid there looking up at the ceiling feeling very proud of myself. "I got him again." and I just smirked.

A few moments passed an in walked Dr. Merrick. "Ms. Ayer, I must request that you do not say another word until this procedure is over with."

"Alright Dr., whatever you say." I turned my head as not to look at him and the procedure continued. I could hear the machine clicking and turning. I believe that it must of took twenty or more different angle pictures of my body and then it was done. The nurse handed me some towels and told me I could go into the ladies room and clean myself. I thanked her and got down from the table holding the towels between my legs. Not a pretty picture, but I did make it to the ladies room without any accidental leakage. I left the ladies room and headed for the locker room.

It was while I was walking that I heard the doctors voice. "Ms Ayer would you come over to my office when you are dressed please. I would like to speak to you." It was Dr. Merrick's voice.

Oh brother, I am in trouble now. But I continued on my way to the locker room and changed my clothes. I walked through the hallway passing some of the nurses that had been in the exam room with me. All I got from them were smiles.

I knocked on Dr. Merrick's office door and heard, "Come in Ms. Ayer." When I opened the door he was sitting at his desk. A big smile took over his face as I walked toward him. "You really caught me off guard this morning young lady."

"I apologize Dr Merrick. I don't know where that statement came from," I confessed.

"I do, you're a very funny lady with a wonderful sense of humor," he admitted. But I wanted you to know that I am going to use you as the first patient for my new radiation machine. This machine will eliminate the need for you to be admitted into the hospital for internal radiation treatments. It can all be done right here, if that is acceptable to you?"

"Of course Dr. Merrick, I have total confidence in your opinion. When will I start receiving radiation from the new machine?"

"It won't be for a couple of weeks. We are not totally set up and this machine is used at the very end of your scheduled treatments. But it will add about two additional weeks of treatment. I feel that this new machine will enhance your chances to be cancer free."

"Alright Doctor," I said.

"One more thing, Ms. Ayer," he added. Try and behave yourself."

"I will give it my best shot," I said smiling. He stood up and shook my hand and I turned and walked out of his office with a big smile on my face. It seemed as if everyone in the building had heard about my little comment, as everyone that passed me was still smiling. I smiled back and was happy that I made them all a little happier in such an unhappy environment I stepped outside and there was Sue sitting in her car. She raised her arm holding a cup of coffee for me. I waved and walked toward her. I could hardly wait to tell her what a little devil I had been.

Chapter 55
Almost the Finish Line

I was awakened to the sound of howling winds. I slid off my bed and walked to my window. Outside everything was white. I could hardly see the road the snow was coming down so heavily. Today was the last day of February. As usual in New England, February usually brings a serious snow storm, and the way it looked right now I think this was it. By the looks of the depth of the snow it had probably been snowing all night long. I hope my appointment won't be cancelled at the radiation center, I thought. I don't have many more treatments to go and I hate to have one be cancelled. I will just have to wait and see if they call from the doctors office.

My strength was beginning to return and my attitude was upbeat. Just the thought of being so close to the finish was getting through each day. I had been marking off the days on my calender every night before I fell asleep. I still wonder how I have made it this far. I can't remember a lot of the days. My mind won't return them to me. I know those memories are in there, but apparently it is best that I can't remember them for now. Perhaps someday when I least expect it, I will be able to recall the missing hours and days.

Last Thursday, I am ashamed to say, was a terrible day. I sat on Brandon's couch upstairs and flatly refused to go for a treatment. I was crying and carrying on hysterically. Where this hysteria came from I do not know. I just couldn't hold it in any longer even with my morning shower tears. I am still so sore in my lower region, no one can imagine. I am raw sore. Even the shower water hitting me, hurts, and Dr. Merrick does not want me to take baths. Brandon tried buying a new shower head. He removed the old one with the hopes that this new one would release softer burst of water spray. But it truly didn't make much of a difference even though I told Brandon, I thought that the new shower head helped. He had gone to so much trouble and the expense of this new shower spray was not something that we could afford. Anyway, that morning when I fell apart and refused to move off the couch, it was Brandon who took over. "Mom, don't give me any shit!" he stated. I think that is the first time my son ever swore at me in his life. "Your going if I have to carry you. So get your coat." It was then that I saw that Alex and little Bri were getting hysterical themselves. They had no idea what was going on. The both began to yell at their father and tugging at his shirt and pants.

"You leave Meme alone," Alex cried.

It was at that point that I snapped out of my stubborn streak and my crying. I was devastated to think that I had frightened the girls so. I immediately calmed down and called the girls to me. Bran stepped back and sat at the kitchen table.

"Your Daddy is right. He is not being mean to me. It's Meme who was being very bad this morning. You see, I have to go to the doctors every single day or the doctors won't be able to kill all the bad cancer in my body. I am so sorry that I was being bad. My only excuse is that sometimes I feel so very sick that I don't think I can be brave enough to withstand another treatment. Can you understand what I am trying to explain to you?" I asked. Both Alex and Bri nodded their heads yes. "Your Daddy would never ever be mean to me. He only wants me to get well, and he knows that my going for treatments will make me better. So please don't cry anymore and please tell your Daddy that you are sorry, and I will too."

Alex put her arms around me and gave me a kiss quickly followed by Bri. Then they both walked over to their father and said, "I'm sorry daddy."

I followed them and hugged my son and also said, "I'm sorry Bran." Needless to say, I will never have another outburst such as that ever again. No matter how badly I am hurting.

Today, I will be the first patient to receive radiation from the "new machine." I had talked to the nurses and Dr. Merrick attempting to learn further information regarding any new side effects this machine might cause. But the answer was always the same, "No, you should not feel any differently at all." I shall keep my fingers crossed on that statement.

I heard the phone ringing upstairs which told me it was most likely from the doctors office. I walked as quickly as I could to the bottom of the stairs and listened. I could hear Sue say, "Alright, thank you."

"Did they cancel my appointment?"

"No, the receptionist said some of the employees were already there, it was up to you whether you wanted to go in or not. Do you want to go Pam?"

"If you wouldn't mind driving in this stuff? I hate the thought of missing an appointment."

"Don't worry about the snow, your doctor is only around the corner from here. So get yourself ready and we will go."

"Oh thank you Sue." I said. I can be dressed in a flash."

The new machine was placed in a brand new room which had been under construction since I started my first treatments. I assume the newly constructed room was build especially for the purpose of holding this new machine. The machine was smaller than I thought it would be. I don't know what I expected, but it looked less intimidating than I had mentally pictured. It sat there, just waiting for me. I had both of the nurse's laughing as I go onto the table. I asked, "Has this new gizmo been tested or am I going to be fried like a piece of chicken?"

Mary giggled until she had tears in her eyes. "Your guess is as good as ours," she replied still giggling.

Theresa got into the giggles adding, "You wouldn't make much of a meal, not enough meat on you." The three of us were still laughing when Dr. Merrick walked in.

"I always know where you are, Ms Ayer. Can you behave yourself this morning so this new machine can do it's work?" he asked with a smile.

"Oh yes sir. I'll be as quiet as a mouse."

"Just lie down Ms. Ayer and be serious. Let this fantastic machine do what it does best."

The treatment was over quickly. The new machine moved back into the starting position and became silent. "Am I done?" I asked Dr. Merrick.

"Yes young lady your finished. How was it?"he asked.

"Fast" I answered. Your all set for today then," he replied. Drive home safely in this bad weather."

I told Theresa I was very thankful for the new machine as I swung my legs over the side of the table. "If it wasn't for this machine, I would be in the hospital with some metal type of object stuck inside me for a few days. Not something I would be enjoying I am sure of that.

"Are you sure of that?" Theresa asked laughing.

"Oh you bad girl" I said giggling. I was still laughing when I went to leave the room. I said my goodbyes and went to the locker room and got dressed and quickly headed for the front door of the building.

Sue and the kids were parked in the almost empty parking lot. The snow was still coming down. I guess there is no school today. Thank goodness I didn't have to miss my appointment. The receptionist sitting at the desk informed me just as I was walking by her that I should call ahead regarding tomorrow's appointment. Just in case the storm continued through the day and night. Apparently she was cancelling all of the afternoon appointments for the rest of the day.

Naturally the girls were wound up with excitement regarding the snow and no school. We had been lucky so far this winter and snow had been scarce for this part of New England. The girls were dressed and ready to make their first snowman of the year.

I watched them from the living room window. They both were rolling around and making snow angels. Try as they may, the snowman was not cooperating. Unfortunately the snow was too powdery for the production of a snowman. But they refused to come in. They looked like snowmen themselves. Their little faces were a bright pink and their eyes were sparkling. I yelled out the front door and said, " Why don't you try and shovel the driveway to help your Dad?"

"We don't have a shovel," Alex replied.

"You don't need a shovel, I will get you the broom." I pulled a broom out of the kitchen closet and handed it to Alex who was waiting at the door. She looked totally confused.

"Daddy always uses a shovel." she said questioningly.

"Try it Alex."

"The broom will work fine."

She gave the snow a sweep and saw how easily the snow moved. "This is great Meme!" "Daddy will be so surprised when he gets home." She immediately began sweeping the driveway and the steps. Alex was always a little helper. Bri was just to busy having fun. She continued rolling around and jumping into the fresh snow.

When the two of them finally came in the house they looked like two frozen popsicles. They were covered with snow and soaking wet. Sue sputtered about getting the rug all wet, and for them to get out of those wet clothes immediately. But she was smiling while she assisted them in undressing.

Today had been a good day. Watching the girls play in the snow made me think of my own children playing in much happier times. But I won't be sad today. Not today. I am almost finished with my treatments.

Chapter 56
The Surprise

This is it. Today is the day! The day I have been waiting for all these months. I can hardly believe that I have actually made it. The past few days have dragged so much I thought I would drive myself crazy. Now it's 6:00 a.m., and I am sitting here fully dressed watching the clock. I don't think I slept more than an hour or two all night long. I watched television until my eyes hurt. I tried taking a "Xanax," and an "Ambien" but neither one of them worked. I guess I was just too excited about today. I would guess that it was exhaustion that finally put me to sleep.

My usual morning shower held no tears for me this morning. Instead I got on my knees in the tub and thanked the Lord for being with me on this long journey. I just stayed there and let the water fall on me while I continued my conversation with God. I can honestly say that I did not feel any pain as the soap and water hit my vulnerable spots. I just continued thanking God.

I took extra effort this morning with my make-up and my hair (yes, I still have all my hair). Today I was going to say good bye to some very nice people. I will miss my conversations with my new friends, but not the treatments. I shared a lot of my thoughts with the ladies. Thoughts that only they could understand. We truly got to know a lot about each other. And we certainly had a lot of laughs. I know that sounds strange under the circumstances, but we really did laugh. Sometimes there is nothing else to do but laugh.

While upstairs I had made myself some coffee, and was sitting with the cup in my hand when Brandon and Sue came out of their bedroom.

"What's the matter Mom?" "Can't sleep?" Brandon asked.

"I am so nervous and excited I can hardly stand it.

"Would you like something to eat this morning before you go?" Sue asked.

"I really would. I am hungry, but I don't dare. I don't want to take the chance of being sick to my stomach because I am so nervous. But thank you Sue."

Brandon asked, "Are you actually having a treatment this morning?"

"I am really not sure what is going to happen this morning. I don't know what to expect. I will just have to wait and see." The next hour passed very slowly.

Alex and Bri got up and they were as excited as I was about the end of my treatments. "This means your all better and you don't have any more cancer?" Bri asked.

"You know Bri, you are absolutely right. I don't have any more cancer." I had been so busy thinking about only the treatments, I hadn't thought of the fact that I would be cancer free. I would be an official "Cancer Survivor." Today is truly a day for a celebration.

At last it was time to leave. I hugged the girls and my son. "I'll be home in a little while." I said smiling.

"We'll be waiting for you," Brandon replied.

Sue was very quiet on the drive to the doctors. "Is there anything wrong Sue?" I asked.

"Pam I am just so happy. We have all been so scared during your illness. I have had some very bad times with Brandon that you knew nothing about. He was scared to death that he was going to lose you, we all were. He cried at night sometimes so hard that I thought he was going to die from fear of losing you."

"There will be no more tears from today. We may be broke, but we are finally healthy. I have to believe that all this happened for a reason, and things are going to improve." I gave her a hug before I got out of the car. "I don't know what I would have done without you, Brandon, Rah, and Jay."

"I would have never made it without my family having been by my side through this."

Sue smiled and said, "I am going to go and get a box of doughnuts and we will celebrate when I pick you up. Do you think you will be in there long this morning?"

"Sue, I really don't know."

"Don't worry about it, I will be here when you come out," she said smiling.

"Good Luck"

I stepped out of the car and started walking toward the building. If I never see this building again, I won't care. It seems like I have spent a lifetime in here. So many days, so much fear and pain. I opened the door and walked into the reception area. A nurse was standing talking to the receptionist when I came inside. "Ms. Ayer, Dr. Merrick wants you to go into the first exam room on the right."

"He will be with you shortly."

I smiled and walked directly toward the exam room. There was a dressing gown placed on the chair next to the exam table. I automatically undressed and sat on the table. A few minutes passed and I heard a knock at the door.

"Are you dressed?' It was Dr. Merrick's voice.

"Yes, I am dressed."

He walked in with a big smile on his face. "Well young lady this is your last eternal exam. I bet your happy about that?"

"You can't imagine," I answered with a big smile.

He examined me quickly and said simply, "Everything looks great. Congratulations young lady!"

I smiled and said a simply "thank you doctor."

"You can get dressed now, I will be right back." He turned and left the room. I immediately got off the table, and dressed and sat in the chair and waited.

I heard another knock at the door. "Are you dressed?"

"Yes, you can come in." He walked in only this time the door was left open.

As he walked in the door he was smiling, but he was holding a small white box. At first I thought perhaps it was some new cream he was giving me for my condition. But he handed me the box without saying a word.

"What's this?" I asked.

"Ms. Ayer, as you know we were extremely successful in shrinking your tumor. But the radiation also shrunk some of the surrounding area as well. You are an extremely small built woman and even with the accuracy of the radiation beams other areas were effected." I looked at him and was at a total loss regarding what he was talking about. "Let me show you what I am talking about." He opened the box and pulled out an object. It was white and about six inches long. It resembled a candle. "Think of this as a prescription. It should be inserted once a day and kept inside you for at least ten minutes. In time it will stretch your vagina. You should use this every day. Your vagina has been severely altered by the radiation, this instrument should help in assisting you to regain a somewhat normal sex life." Then he smiled a very wide smile. "My advice to you is when you start dating again, only date very small men." It was at that point what he had been explaining to me made sense.

"Doctor, am I that small inside? "

"Yes, young lady you are." I sat back down in the chair not saying a word. This information had come out of no where. I had never even thought about such a thing occurring in my body. I don't why. It does make perfect sense. I just wasn't prepared for it. I didn't know whether to laugh or to cry. I sat there for a minute and said nothing. I then stood up and shook Dr. Merrick's hand. "It's a small price to pay for my life. Get it? I said with a wide smile. Thank you for everything doctor. "

"You have a wonderful life, Ms. Ayer," he said. Then he turned and walked out the door. I stood there holding the little white box for a few minutes, and then carefully placed it into my pocketbook. I gathered up my coat and purse and walked out of the exam room and began looking for my two friends. I didn't have to walk far when I saw the two of them standing around the next corner talking. Theresa saw me first. She smiled immediately and started walking toward me. Mary was right behind her. We hugged and I thanked them for their friendship. I tried to tell them both how much their kindness had meant to me, but my eyes began to fill with tears. So, I just hugged them both one more time and said good bye. I walked the corridor for one more time heading for the front door. "Good bye," I said to the receptionist and I opened the door and walked outside. I immediately saw Sue sitting in her car with the motor running.

I didn't walk to the car, I ran. It was over.

Chapter 57
My New Beginning

I opened the door of Sue's car and sat down on the front seat and began to cry. I cried with tears of joy. I just could not believe that it was finally over, and that I had survived. Sue put her arms around me, and we both sat there and continued crying. When I had at last got a grip on my emotions I told Sue, "We have to go home, I have to call Rah and everyone else."

First I called my Mom and Dad. I was so excited that my Mom had a difficult time understanding me. "I'm all through Mom."

"What do you mean your all through?" she asked.

"With the treatments. Today was my last day. I am speaking to you cancer free."

"Oh my God," she exclaimed. Dick, Pam is all through with her treatments and she is cured."

I could hear Dad in the background but I couldn't understand what he was saying. "I have to call Rah and Jay now. I will talk to you later on today. Bye Mom, I love you."

Rah was next on my list. She must have been expecting to hear from me as the phone rang only once. "Rah, I am done. I'm going to live."

"Oh Mom, I have been praying so hard for you. I knew that you would not leave me."

"I love you Rah, and I want to thank you for all you have done for me in the past eight months. I could not have done it without you. I have to call Jay now. I will talk to you later."

Ann answered the phone and I immediately started laughing and trying to get the words out. "No more treatments. I am cured. Is Jay home?

"No he is at work, but I will tell him just as soon as he gets home. That's wonderful news. He will be so relieved. He has been very scared regarding your cancer."

"I know, but it is alright now. I have to go and calm myself down, but I just had to let everyone know the good news. Please have Jay call me."

"Don't worry Pam, he will call you as fast as he hears the news."

My last phone call was to my brother. I dialed his cell phone number that he had given me months before. "Hello?' he said.

"This is your cancer free sister speaking," I said proudly.

There was a short pause and then "Pam?"

"Yes you silly goose, how many sisters do you have?"

"Your all done, and they got it all? Yes they did Edward. Today was my last treatment and the doctor examined me and sent me away with a clean bill of health. I just wanted to let you know and tell you that I love you very much."

"I love you to little sister. How is everything else going for you?"he asked.

"Oh the usual, but I am getting by. Don't worry about me. I am going to start living again. Is Fern home? No, she is working, but I will give her the good news when she gets home."

"Well, you take care dear brother and I will be talking to you again real soon.

I have got to calm myself down before I have a heart attack. Bye for now, and remember I love you."

"Bye little sister and congratulations."

I walked downstairs and went into my bedroom. I got down on my knees and thanked God with all my heart. "Please God, let me do something good with my life starting today" I prayed. "Help me to be the person that you want me to be. Guide me and never let me forget what I have been through all these months. Thank you for my family. Without you and them, I would have never had the strength."

As I sit here typing the story of my fight with cancer, it is as close to the truth as I can remember. There are still a lot of blank days that I believe are lost forever. However, it is now five years later and I am still cancer free. I met a wonderful man who is kind and gentle. I love him very much and I am now residing in Texas with him. My daughter Rah has moved here with her family to start a new life as I have. Unfortunately, Bran and Sue are now divorced. Jay and his wife Ann had a new baby yesterday. Jason now has a brand new son. My granddaughter Amanda has given me two great grandchildren, both boys. The oldest is Jonathan and the newest edition is 5 months old and his name is Anthony. My Mom and Dad are both alive and well and as busy as ever. I retired from the Post Office and have never looked back. My dear brother is still traveling the world with his wife Fern and I had the chance to see him just a couple of months ago in Texas. My beautiful grandchildren are just that. They have grown up to be lovely young ladies and little Kyle (name) just had a birthday today. He is nine years old. As for my ex, he is still alive and as miserable as he deserves to be.

I have tried to learn from my cancer experience and recalling all these memories has been very difficult for me. But God and I are still very good friends, and I still talk to him daily. I still thank him every day for all the blessings he has given me throughout my life. I hope that my story will help someone with a battle that they might be fighting. I am in no way a doctor and I don't possess any type of degree, but my simple advise is never give up and love the people in your lives for tomorrow, they may be gone.

I wish to thank my children for supporting me and loving me. Without them, I would not have been able to survive. And to my friend, the southern bell, I will think about you tomorrow, when I take my shower without any tears.

Printed in the United States
31035LVS00002B/197